Nine Easy Steps To Complete Health & Well Being

A Physician's guide to Health, Happiness & Vitality

by

B. Singh, MD

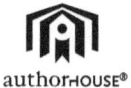

AuthorHouse™
1663 Liberty Drive, Suite 200
Bloomington, IN 47403
www.authorhouse.com
Phone: 1-800-839-8640

First published by AuthorHouse 2/28/2008

ISBN: 978-1-4343-3020-8 (sc)
ISBN: 978-1-4343-3664-4 (hc)

Library of Congress Control Number: 2007906064

Printed in the United States of America
Bloomington, Indiana

This book is printed on acid-free paper.

"A man should look for what is, and not for what he thinks should be"
                              ~Albert Einstein

Contents

With deep gratitude to :

The Supreme Power for helping me realize that
The greatest treasures are
Happiness, Health and Love

My parents who have taught me to
Be Happy, Work faithfully and Love all

And my husband and children
who have shown me how to
Live and Enjoy every moment

Introduction

About 4.6 billion years ago, as the gases in the universe forming the "solar nebula" settled in to form the star we call the sun and its solar system, neither the collective universe nor any other atom had a clue of what was coming. A billion years later, perhaps as a result of elements essential for life being brought to earth by meteorites, life began to take form on earth. And yet, it was only 200,000 years ago that the first *Homo sapiens*, a species called man, walked the earth. Nature sure has taken its time in making man, and the progress that this species has made is phenomenal. Man continues to amaze the universe and himself with his achievements.

And yet, after developing from the Stone Age to the Jet Age, the most desirous achievements of a lifetime are still good health, happiness, inner peace, and true love. Money, success, and fame can only provide monetary and momentary comforts, feelings of elation, and time-limited pleasure. The cyclical pattern of these materialistic, ego-boosting elements brings with it stress, depression, and frustration as the intensity or availability of its elements fades. On the other hand, a person who has good health, mental peace, and spiritual satisfaction does not need any external stimulus to feel good and happy.

A study published in the February 2007 issue of *Psychological Sciences* that was conducted by Harvard psychologists confirms the importance of educating the mind of undertakings that will positively impact health. Just by so doing, one can improve his or her health and well-being. This was shown in a comparison between a group of workers who were made aware of the healthy aspects of their activities and another group who were oblivious to this, even though both the groups were undertaking the same workload.

As we rejuvenate our bodies, open our minds, and connect with the limitless potential energy of the universe, we begin to receive whatever we desire from the abundance of the universe. In this state of complete well-being, as we harmonize our energies with those of the universe, our needs and desires easily manifest.

> *"Happiness is not something ready made. It comes from your own actions".*
>
> ~Dalai Lama

During my years at medical school, I was taught that physical, mental, and spiritual health are essential and that they intermingle to create a state of well-being within an individual. The attainment of that state is a prerequisite to a healthy and happy existence. I did not understand the true meaning of this until I stepped out into the real world and started my own family. When I had to lose fifty pounds after the birth of our third child; when I had to balance the mental challenges of attending to the needs of my profession as a medical intensivist with the demands of my family; and when, despite all materialistic comforts and professional progress, I strived for peace within; the true meaning of complete health and its practical applications dawned on me.

My quest for knowledge on physical, mental, and spiritual health started in my teenage years, and for thirty years now my passion for progress in this area has led me to learn from the research in science, the philosophy and wisdom of great men and women, and most importantly, lessons from life experiences and intuitive knowledge. This has allowed me to pursue the attainment of complete well-being with devotion. Through all this, I have kept in mind one guiding principle that was ingrained in me by my father:

> *"A problem is not the problem; not finding a solution is the problem."*

I dedicate this book to my family, who have taught me that one of the greatest comforts of life is in loving and belonging; to my teachers, who have shown me that one of the greatest joys of life is in learning and understanding; and to my patients, who have enlightened me by showing me that the greatest peace comes from caring and healing.

In our desire for materialistic gains and our efforts to provide for our families and seek advantageous positions, we have left this concept far behind. The result is before us: increasing rates of obesity, heart diseases, and stroke; astoundingly high incidences of depression, suicide, and homicide; and widespread unethical and immoral behavior. This book is a sincere effort to put forth in easy steps a recipe for complete well-being that will allow one to feel well, perform well, and look well. As long as one demonstrates determination, discipline, and devotion, success is sure to follow. May we all be blessed with complete health and well-being.

"He has achieved success who has lived well, laughed often, and loved much"
~Bessie Stanley

Preface

Nature has endowed each one of us with a complete blueprint for survival, progress, and harmony. The basic intent of every organism is to exist in a synchronized state with itself and its surroundings. And yet, how often do we feel that way? We all want to achieve a state of complete well-being. Maybe we even want to live the maximum possible livable age (Jeanne Calment of France, 1875–1997, lived 122 years and 164 days) while retaining vitality, vigor, fun, frolic, and peace!

The very fact that you have obtained and are reading this book is a testimony to your desire. But why do we read book after book and article after article and yet feel like we are only looking at pieces of a puzzle? Because we are! There are various aspects of health that are as intermingled as the different threads woven together to make a colorful garment. It is the intent of this book to give the reader a broad approach to health with attention to details while offering easy, practical ways to apply this information to a challenging lifestyle.

It is imperative to discuss another issue at the outset—our achievements. Despite our best intentions and desires, why are we unable to reach our goals? What good will it serve us if we have reached the last page without having made any positive strides toward achieving a feeling of well-being? If we feel lacking in health, let it be a good reason to change the situation.

> "In order to change we must be sick and tired of being sick and tired."
>
> ~Anonymous

However, if the contents of this book are to be of any benefit to us, it is recommended that we follow the simple rules of achievement.

Desire and Intent

Before any goal can be achieved, it is essential that the individual has a sincere desire to reach it. You have already demonstrated this by obtaining and reading this book!

Knowledge and Understanding

Humans are unique in the degree of development of their comprehensive capabilities. One may read or obtain information about any issue, but unless it is assimilated, it does not become knowledge. Once we have acquired knowledge, it is imperative that we understand it and apply it in our lives according to our needs. What is provided in this book is information, so it is up to each one of us to understand the contents and convert it to knowledge. It will help if only one section is read at a time. If needed, revisit these sections to enhance memory and understanding. Before starting on another section, it is crucial to apply that information in order to reap the benefits.

Planning and Execution

No two humans function or think alike; neither do they have the exact same schedule. The information presented here can be applied to all individuals, but not necessarily in the same order of importance. Knowing our own weaknesses, needs, and lifestyles, we should plan to incorporate the suggestions in an order most suitable to us. Good planning is half the work. However, execution is equally important.

Procrastination never helps. As you learn a helpful skill, it is important to implement it to see the benefits. Many people buy plenty of health books, subscribe to a few health magazines, and think they are on their road to healing. If it makes one feel good, that is fine, but it is like keeping seeds in your pocket and hoping to see a tree grow from them someday! Just plant them and the miracle starts! The growth of a seed into a tree is truly amazing, but it becomes a reality only when the seed is appropriately nurtured. Take the first step, and the rest will be easy strides.

Analysis and Correction

It is as important to monitor one's actions and set intervals for the analysis of goals and results as it is to put forth effort. If things are not working out the way they should, ask yourself: did our intent change, did our desire weaken, did our knowledge and understanding not hold up, did our planning fail, or did our actions fall short of what was desired? Putting checkpoints in place and having appropriate correctional measures ready will help us to continue on the right path; this goes a long way in ensuring success.

In Summary: Attain, Retain, and Maintain.

It will serve us well to keep in mind that good health and well-being do not relate only to increasing the number of years that we exist in a mortal form, but also to feeling well each day of our life—and thereafter!

> *Always remember that quick fixes only give short-term results. For lifelong health and well-being, one has to implement the right lifestyle.*

Every human being is the author of his own health or disease.

~Buddha

Overview

"Thousands upon thousands of persons have studied disease. Almost no one has studied health."
~Adelle Davis

Health is often looked at as a freedom from disease (*dis-ease: not at ease*) or a sound state of existence. But the complete potential of this state is actually a harmonious, blissful, peaceful, gratifying, glorious, and rejuvenating form of well-being. No formula can claim to get you there. Just as there are many roads to get us to our homes, there are many routes to attaining this state of complete well-being. Regardless of what path one takes, it is important to remember that the needs of a human being are not merely physical. These needs are not even satisfied with psychological or social achievements. Unless we also attend to the third dimension of our health—the needs of our soul—we cannot enjoy complete health.

"A healthy body is the guest-chamber of the soul; a sick, its prison."
~Francis Bacon

It has taken millions of years of evolution from the time of the first primates—the ancestors of humans—to form the *Homo sapiens*. This species, *Homo sapiens* (popularly referred to as humans), has probably evolved beyond the imaginations of its creators. No other known living animal has the traits exemplified by humans that have allowed us humans to raise their average life expectancy by twenty-five years within a century. Its unique physical structure as the only mammal to be completely mobile on two limbs, its capability to oppose the thumb to its fingers, and its lack of adequate natural fur have allowed it to be creative and alter its physical surroundings. Its intelligence, its language development (both in the spoken and sign form), its learning capabilities, its memory, and its reasoning skills have allowed it to create a whole new world for itself. And yet its feelings, emotions, and abilities to comprehend and distinguish love and fear have kept it wrapped up in mental acrobatics. Its insight and intuitive nature, combined with its superior mental capabilities, have allowed it to perceive the unseen, recognize hidden powers, and experience supernatural forces, as has been described by spiritually evolved individuals, such as Mother Theresa, Mahatma Gandhi, and Paramahansa Yogananda.

How then can attainment of health, happiness, and harmony be possible with attention to just the physical aspect of existence? Indeed, we need to address and satisfy all those metaphysical issues if success has to be achieved. And yet, it needs to be done simply to allow us the benefit of complete understanding and easy practice. *Nine Easy Steps for Complete Health and Well-being* is a blend of modern science and traditional philosophy, sprinkled with the wisdom of great men and women of honor. It is an in-depth analysis of how to respect the body, use and transcend the mind, and bask in the luminous glow of the spirit by connecting with the eternal universal power, which is a state that is natural to the soul, yet often oblivious to our minds.

Basic Concepts

Our health has three basic components: physical, mental, and spiritual. Although each of these aspects is multidimensional, it will serve us well to see them under some broad headings, as those symbolizing body, mind, and spirit. The external manifestation of the body is seen as the physique, the mind shows itself as temperament and personality, and the soul shines forth as the character of the individual.

The following diagram is intended to visually simplify each component of health and its attributes. It would be worthwhile to study the diagram to comprehend the influence of each of the nine essential components contributing to health.

Mind

1. Attitude
2. Thoughts and Habits
3. Stress

Body

4. Nutrition
5. Activity
6. Rest

Soul

7. Supreme Power
8. Self
9. Laws of Nature

The Journey

"There's lots of people who spend so much time watching their health, they haven't time to enjoy it."
~Josh Billing

When we plant a seed and nourish it day after day, the joy of watching it grow is its own reward. If we were just waiting for it to grow into a big tree and give fruits, we would be missing a wonderful opportunity to marvel at nature, learn, understand, and rejoice in miracles. Each day should bring a joyous realization of the wonders of life. As the stems appear, as the leaves show up, as the plants grow, and as the flowers and fruits emerge, we should be thankful for the miracle of life.

As you begin your joyful journey into the fascinating world of your body, mind, and soul, remember that this journey should be as enjoyable as reaching the destination of complete health and well-being. This should not be considered a task or as another duty or zealous desire. It should be considered a way of life, a wonderful gift of realization that existence can be simple, easy, fun, and yet fulfilling.

In order to enhance understanding, an attempt has been made to simplify the intricate, interdependent, and complicated issues pertaining to health. For this reason, physical, mental, and spiritual aspects of health have been categorized under separate headings. However, no aspect of health and well-being stands alone. Each is intimately connected to the other aspects in both obvious and hidden ways. Concerns of the mind easily affect our physical state, the spiritual state of an individual influences the mental attitudes and functioning, the physical health of the body can alter our mental capacities, and so on and so forth. Nevertheless, discussing these issues in separate sections does not take away their interdependence. There are facets of health that have indistinct boundaries, and their discussion overlaps in different sections of the text.

We should always keep in mind that we are intended by nature to exist in a state of complete well-being every moment that we are alive; we just have to discover it.

> *"It is more important to add life to your years than years to your life."*
>
> ~ Anonymous

Part 1

Essentials for Health and Well-being

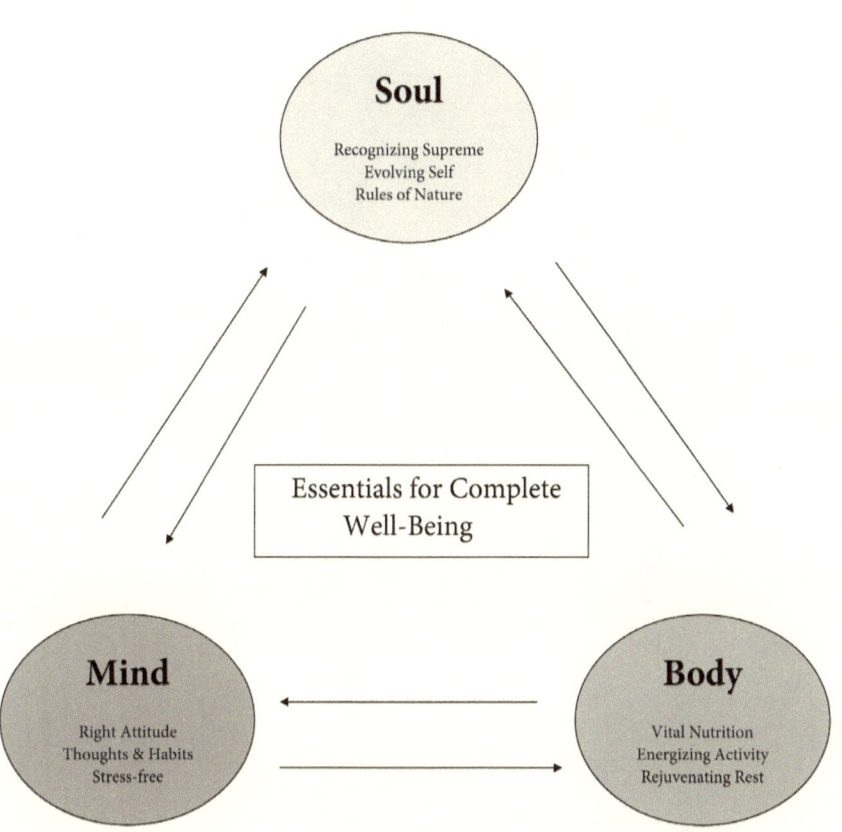

Soul

Recognizing Supreme
Evolving Self
Rules of Nature

Essentials for Complete
Well-Being

Mind

Right Attitude
Thoughts & Habits
Stress-free

Body

Vital Nutrition
Energizing Activity
Rejuvenating Rest

Mind

"'Tis the mind that makes the body rich."
~William Shakespeare

If we think for just a moment about what we would be without our minds, we suddenly realize that we would cease to exist! All our perceptions of self and others, our thoughts, our feelings, our emotions, and our behaviors conjure up images, either real or imagined. These and innumerable other functions that our mind performs bring forth the flavors of life. Mind is to the body as aroma is to the flower, as warmth is to the sunshine. Its complexities perplex us; its manifest, or conscious, aspect amazes us; and its hidden, or unconscious, part confuses us. And yet "we" would become nonexistent without it.

Mind, as described by Webster's dictionary, is the part of an individual that feels, perceives, thinks, wills, and reasons. If we try to understand it and tame it, we can be our own masters, reaching new heights in our achievements, relationships, and inner contentment. But if we let it take us for a ride, we may never reach our intended destination. Understanding three simple attributes of the mind's function can help us feel well, perform well, and achieve the progress that we desire. Simply put, these are:

- Attaining and Maintaining the Right Attitude

- Developing Progressive Thoughts and Habits

- Keeping the Mind Stress Free

Right Attitude

Chapter 1

Attitude

"The happiest people are those who seem to have no particular reason for being happy except that they are so"
~William Inge

Probably no other aspect of our lives has more impact on our thoughts, emotions, behaviors, and actions, than our outlook on life. Two people may go through the exact same experience, and yet they can have two completely different outcomes. What prompts their thoughts, moods, drive to achieve, desire to overcome obstacles, and ability to remain content with the outcome are their dispositions toward a situation. Whether we are in harmony with our surroundings, happy with our relationships, or at peace with ourselves is a reflection of our frame of mind. This perception of our experiences is what we refer to as *attitude.*

A couple of years ago, the amazing power of attitude on health was reported and scientifically supported in BBC News.[1] Studies led by Dr. Glen Ostir of the University of Texas led him to conclude that attitude had positive effects on physical and mental health. Similarly, Professor Thomas Hess of North Carolina State University showed improved memory performance in older adults who were primed by positive words describing ageing i.e., "positive stereotyping". It is speculated that positive attitude may directly affect health by altering the chemical balance of the body and possibly affecting the immune system. Additionally, it may help to boost a person's health by making

---

[1] URL- http://news.bbc.co.uk/2/hi/health/3642356.stm

it more likely that he or she will be successful in life. Therefore, it is definitely worth exploring our attitude further.

In a broader sense, an individual either has a positive outlook, referred to as an optimist, or he or she has a negative attitude, an individual who is prototyped as a pessimist. A certain type of outlook may be inherent to the nature of an individual, or it may be circumstantial. In the latter of the two, regardless of the kind of experience, an individual always tends to consistently react either positively or negatively each time a certain situation occurs. For example, say a group of friends want to go out water-skiing. Despite everyone else's agreement, one of them does not want to do that. His friends accuse him of being a spoilsport, but on closer questioning, they discover that his brother had a serious water-skiing accident during one of his outings. This would be a circumstantial outlook.

On the other hand, there are individuals who are always complaining about something or the other, criticizing people for their behavior even when they mean well, finding faults with their jobs even when they are sought-after positions, missing opportunities because they feel there are unseen dangers, etc. Essentially, they are moving around with gray glasses on all the time! If only they could take off their glasses and start looking at the brighter side of things, they would suddenly open up a whole new world of possibilities.

It is indeed within our power to choose optimism or pessimism. What are we to gain with pessimism? Gloom, hopelessness, depression, and missed opportunities. What are we to lose? Cheerfulness, opportunities, and motivation. If you were dying of hunger and someone brought you a donut, you could start complaining that instead of being given a full snack, you have been offered a baked good with 50 percent cut out in the center! On the other hand, you could gratefully and graciously accept the offering, complementing the interesting shape that has allowed the donut to be baked to perfection! This is pessimism versus optimism!

Regardless of the situation we are in, an optimistic mind allows us to look at the bright side of an issue. It does not allow external influences to cloud it with fear, and it keeps its light burning with a never-ending flame of hope and happiness. By doing so, it maintains the clarity of its psyche, keeps its analytic skills awake, and sharpens its reasoning power, despite adversities. By keeping its presence of mind, it is able to work toward options and solutions instead of descending into regret and dismay. As correctly depicted in the classic *Paradise Lost*:

> *The mind is its own place, and in itself can make heav'n of hell, a hell of heav'n.*
> ~John Milton

There may be circumstances in which changing our environment is not possible. An optimistic person is still able to find reasons to stay cheerful and peaceful despite such negative influences. As an example, there are people who feel distressed with winter. Clearly it is not possible to change the weather unless one changes his or her location. In such a situation, an optimist will still be able to find reasons to be happy: taking time to make a snowman with the kids, sledding, enjoying the fireplace, concentrating on indoor sports, and looking forward to some days off from work!

Chapter 2

What Is the Right Attitude?

"Man's real life is happy, chiefly because he is ever expecting that it soon will be so."
~Edgar Allan Poe

If one keeps in mind one simple philosophy of life, one can understand how easy it would be to maintain a healthy outlook. That philosophy is, "Everything in this world is there for a reason, and my role is to do my best and be my best." No one has to pick up blame for anything; there are no regrets and no accusations; there is no digging into the past, and there is no washing dirty laundry in public. Think to yourself, *That is how it turned out; that is what I am going to deal with; and here is what I need and how I need to work with it to achieve the best outcome.* As I have learned from my father, *"A problem is not the problem; not finding a solution is the problem."*

Each thought, each action, each emotion, and each feeling costs us mental energy. We are wasting precious power within ourselves, losing irreplaceable time, and scarring our relationships by harping and continuing to focus on the negative aspects of our experiences. By looking at the positives of a situation, event, or an individual, we are able to appreciate and make amends instead of feeling dejected, dismayed, frustrated, and overwhelmed.

Try this simple experiment next time: approach a friend with faults that you would like him or her to correct, and watch his or her reaction. A person will immediately become defensive, try to deny or justify his or her actions, dislike you for being insensitive, or find your faults and tell you what he or she thinks about you! So the exercise was not only futile, (the person essentially shut themselves down to your suggestions), but you also helped generate a lot of destructive heat, you felt drained by the experience, and you probably lost a good friend. Well, now try telling a friend about some of the qualities that make you like him or her. Then gradually introduce your perception about a particular event and explain why you could not understand what prompted that person to act a certain way during that event. Most of the time, the other individual will start reflecting on the event with you and admit he or she was not comfortable with the way he or she handled the situation. By doing this, your attitude has allowed you to act in a manner that has helped generate an understanding, a resolution of dispute, and a strengthening of your relationship with a good friend. It is nothing but a win-win solution!

Some philosophers recommend that we try to maintain a neutral attitude—an attitude that is neither positive and nor negative, but rather one that is without personal reactions, like that of an observer or a bystander. This philosophy is derived from one of the most ancient religious texts, the Bhagavad Gita. It also forms the underlying principle in the teachings of Lord Buddha, which are promoted as the Path to Nirvana (or Liberation). This is not an easy state to achieve, although the mental energies are probably most preserved by doing this. An individual who practices this technique is able to feel content in most situations and does not feel overwhelmed or unsettled by events and interactions. This is an advanced mental exercise that often calls upon enhanced spiritual strength. With practice hopefully, such strength will be well developed by the time we reach stages of life that require less action and intervention. It is easy to see why grandparents who have achieved this skill are the best people to care for young ones.

We can negatively influence the sensitive development of a small child with our reactions, just as a growing plant may be adversely affected by extremes of the climate. While optimistic reflection can serve as a fertilizer to a growing plant, a neutral attitude can help allow the natural talents of a child to show and grow. It may be worthwhile to explore the application of a neutral or indifferent attitude in matters that are really not within our immediate concern or influence. For example, if an elected politician were found to have some skeletons in his closet, there would be nothing I could do about it. If I wasn't planning to vote for him in the next four-year term anyway, why should I waste my mental resources on the news? No wonder mothers have often told their kids not to talk about politics in public!

What is the ultimate goal to be achieved by having a positive attitude? It appears to be the ability to see every opportunity in our lives as a learning experience rather than a bothersome task, to see every relationship as a precious interaction to cherish or learn from, and to see every event as a test of our strength and a blessing that we are alive to experience. It may be a long road to that achievement, but the ride itself is wonderfully joyous and worth every effort.

Chapter 3

Why Is Attitude So Important?

> "Each of us makes his own weather and determines the
> color of the skies in the emotional universe which he
> inhabits."
>
> ~Fulton J. Sheen

It is a well-described phenomenon in psychology that we can alter our perception of a stimulus by changing our mental disposition. It is much more acceptable to us not to receive an annual raise if we see others getting pay cuts. Similarly, short, sunny days of the still-cold part of spring are welcome after a long winter, while we grumble about the falling temperatures of autumn days after an enjoyable summer.

A person's perception of a stimulus is a function more so of his or her perception than the intensity of the stimulus. We essentially react, act, and feel according to what our senses allow us to perceive due to the influence of our minds. If we have a preconceived notion that there are snakes in the garden, we may jump, shout, or do both if we see a rope. James Allen, in his book *As a Man Thinketh*, has put it very well;

> "Circumstance does not make a man; it reveals him to
> himself."

We are constantly faced with varying situations in our lives that impact our thoughts, feelings, and emotions. Furthermore, our behavior is influenced by how we perceive situations; this thereby affects our actions. Over a period of time, these emotions turn into moods, and moods influence our behavior and actions. Left unaddressed, these become habits, which eventually affect our character, and it is our character that eventually shapes our destiny. In essence, our lives are eventually dictated by our perceptions and our attitudes!

"Weakness of attitude becomes weakness of character."
~Albert Einstein

And it does not stop there! The way in which we receive or approach another individual, interpret his or her ideas and actions, or react to his or her suggestions or advice is more often than not a function of our attitude toward them. Your mother and mother-in-law may make the same suggestion, but coming from one it is advice, while from the other it appears to be interference. Consciously or unconsciously, we allow our perspective toward other individuals to guide our interpretation of our interaction with them. This limits our capacity to enjoy meaningful, enjoyable, and healthy relationships. Unfortunately, it also sometimes robs us of opportunities and prevents us from gaining from another person's experience.

Even small children are intuitively aware of the phenomenon of the effect of attitude on people's lives. I can clearly recall the moment my seven-year-old daughter ran up to me and quizzically asked, "Mommy, do you know what is priceless yet costs nothing?" As I pondered and finally gave her a defeated shake of my head, she grinned and said, "A smile." And indeed, can anyone deny that as a fact? Be it at home or at work, whether we are at the stores or at a gathering, what do we remember the most? What gives us the greatest feeling of comfort and pleasure? To see someone smile at us.

"Every time you smile at someone, it is an action of love, a gift to that person, a beautiful thing."
~Mother Teresa

A smile is a reassurance that we are accepted, that we are welcome, and that we are worthy. It puts us at ease and inspires us to be what we can and achieve what is possible. What if there was a way to transfix this feeling permanently in ourselves? What if we could continuously store within us this feeling of elation, peace, comfort, and confidence? Then we would not need any external influences to modify our development. To me, the way to have the best attitude is to always keep smiling on the inside! As Mahatma Gandhi said,

"You are not fully dressed till you wear your smile."

In essence, modern day research, traditional philosophy, and insight of great minds have come to the same conclusion that the one factor that has been repeatedly shown to have a positive effect on health and longevity is the aspect of positive attitude in an individual. Francis Bacon has put it very well:

To be free minded and cheerfully disposed at hours of meat and sleep and of exercise is one of the best precepts of long lasting."

Chapter 4

The Scientific Basis of Attitude

Feelings of helplessness, fear, and gloom—common accompaniments of pessimism—are actually associated with neuroendocrinal changes within our bodies. Stress hormones such as sympathetic amines and cortisol surge as the body prepares for what has been described as the fright, flight, or fight response. Excitatory neurons that produce emotions of distress and anxiety reverberate, and an individual is caught in a vicious internal cycle of hopelessness. Mental faculties are preoccupied with negative thoughts and concentrate mainly on blame and escape, rather than understanding and learning.

Physical changes are evident, too, such as increased heart rate, higher blood pressure and respiration, wide pupils, tremors, and sweating. Some people may even experience an elevation of body temperature, which is sometimes alluded to as stress fever. Repeated internal imbalances of such a nature are a sure way to rapid aging and an invitation to conditions such as hypertension (high blood pressure) and ischemic cardiac diseases (heart attacks).

On the other hand, a relaxed, cheerful, and peaceful individual tends to have his heart rate, blood pressure, and breathing in normal range. By avoiding accelerations and breakdowns of his systems, he is able to maintain his body in an optimal state of health. Additionally, because of his attitude, he is able to enjoy healthy relationships and supportive groups of friends who act as shock absorbers in times of stress.

The works of scientists like Dr Ronald Grossarth-Maticek have shown that teaching people about positive attitude positively influences health and longevity. In a prospective analysis of longevity after more than a decade of conducting a positive attitude course, he observed that the majority of the people with positive attitudes were still alive, while most of those without were not.

In essence, it cannot be put better than the wise words of Joseph Addison:

> *"Cheerfulness is the best promoter of health and is as friendly to the mind as to the body."*

Man is happy and peaceful by nature, and it is only through a neutral or optimistic view that such a state can be maintained, irrespective of the circumstances. It is worth contemplating why humans would choose to negatively reflect on life situations. This is probably because when we are not fully conscious of our mental state, the mind is easily overcome by basic animal instincts of fright, flight, and fight.

When we first start deflecting our reflections from positive or neutral to negative, our balance of joyful existence is disturbed. This will often play out in our body as signs and symptoms seen in the fright, flight, and fight response. We begin to feel uneasy and restless. If we do not immediately notice and reverse this deflection, the negativity takes over our mind with a strong momentum. This is because the mind starts perceiving the situation as a threat to survival. A continuous stream of negative thoughts overcomes the naturally joyous and peaceful state of our minds and we start feeling depressed. The influences of our past experiences and role models can have similar effects on our thinking.

The situation is not different from a sailing boat that has developed a leak in it. Water quickly rushes in if the leak is not immediately sealed, and the more water rushes in, the heavier the boat gets, and the boat sinks even faster. The solution is to stop the leak in the first place. But how does one attain and maintain the right attitude?

Chapter 5

Attaining and Maintaining the Right Attitude

"I realized the problem was me and nobody could change me except myself."

~John Petworth,

To realize that a healthy attitude is essential to an individual's health and well-being is probably easier than ensuring that we have one! But the realization of what is amiss in our attitude is the first step in the right direction. And as John Petworth has so nobly declared, it is within us to make the difference.

If the right attitude is such a crucial ingredient for good health, are there processes that we can follow to attain, retain, and maintain it? Indeed, it is possible to enjoy this state of positive mental state by using some very simple steps. This can be as simple as A-B-C-D, the essential steps in the right direction:

A: Address yourself
B: Bring in the experts
C: Company you keep
D: Develop your environment

A: Address Yourself

- Are you one of those fortunate people who have the right attitude? An easy way to find out is to note how you feel in the next five situations that you are in. Give yourself a score as per the specifications below:

Agitated	0	Content	1
Restless	0	Relaxed	1
Sad	0	Happy	1

If your score is zero, you are in for the works! If you have a score of two or more, you probably have this health attribute under your belt.

- Start noticing your environment more carefully. Also note the interactions and situations that you are in and carefully analyze the effects they have on your mind. If these effects mainly consist of the states that receive scores of zero, you should question your reactions. Looking at the same scenario from a bystander's perspective and evaluating whether your reactions are justified is crucial to this analysis. Taking the assistance of a close friend with the right attitude can sometimes help you comprehend the situation in times when logic eludes you.

- Thereafter, one should carry on an internal dialogue explaining the futility of negative thoughts. Let your mind race forward and imagine all the possible short- and long-term negative effects that such thoughts could bring. Experience the detrimental physical changes the body is going through, such as restlessness, pounding heart, etc., then perceive the despair and anguish that your mental faculties are experiencing. Realize how draining and exhausting the experience is, and pledge to stop and reverse these effects. As so correctly phrased by the American essayist Edwin Percy Whipple, "*Cheerfulness in most cheerful people is the satisfying result of strenuous discipline.*"

- Whenever you begin to notice negative attitude starting to creep into your reflection, you should stop the thought process by fixing your mind on a physical object or your breath. As you become drawn into negativity, the feeling perpetuates itself like a weed. You become more and more drawn into it because it is compelling and fear inducing, and your mind perceives it as a survival concern. Therefore, consciously diverting your mind until logic prevails is crucial to prevent getting drawn into the whirlpool of negativity.

- Create and migrate into a mental shell of an energized, uplifting, and positive scenario. This may be a vacation spot, a colored wall, a mental picture of a rainbow, a glowing sun, or whatever it is that you identify with positive energy and a happy and peaceful state. (More details on this can be found in the meditation section.) Believe in and strongly implement what you have decided to accomplish.

- Use spiritual strength with the support of faith and hope to enhance and perpetuate the feeling of positive attitude (see discussions under the section on spiritual health).

- Create checkpoints for analyzing your progress, either with yourself or with a close friend who can serve as a good role model. Take a few moments of meditative reflection before meal times to feel the direction of your attitude's energy. Meditating (as discussed under the section on stress) is one of the most effective ways of feeling at ease, gathering positive energy, and enhancing and perpetuating the feeling of contentment. The result is a relaxed, clutter-free, and clear-thinking mind. Just like a picture is depicted better when drawn on a clean sheet of paper than if it is drawn on paper that has already been printed on, the mind is best able to assess and address when it is without a continuous mental dialogue.

B: Bring In the Experts

- The best influences we can allow in our lives are the works and advice of great men and women of honor. What could be easier than reading books or listening to messages from experts on tapes and in seminars? Libraries and bookstores often have these under the sections of mental health, self-help, or psychology.

- Although there is a multitude of material on this subject, my personal literary favorites in this category are *"As a Man Thinketh"* by James Allen, *"Don't Sweat the Small Stuff"* by Richard Carlson, and *"The Power of Now"* by Eckhart Tolle; which are all rich in context and easy in application. Carrying a pocket-sized spiritual book helps me draw on strength at all times.

C: Company You Keep

- As we look around, we find that we are surrounded by all kinds of people with different attitudes. It is also interesting to note that our own reactions are often influenced by what others around us are expressing. Sometimes we unconsciously start echoing the behaviors of our companions. Therefore, it is crucial that we become aware of this possibility and work toward addressing it.

- We should make a conscious effort toward increasing our association and interaction with people who appear to have positive outlooks. On the other hand, individuals who tend to cast doubts regarding outcomes, who spend most of their time criticizing, and who tend to generate anxiety rather than enthusiasm are best avoided (or maybe even given this section to read!).

- We should always remember that we are accountable for our own perspective before we try to influence and correct other people's perspectives. It is, in fact, more time and effort consuming to make other people understand these issues than it is to understand them yourself, and it is also much less satisfying. As we are progressing in the development of the right attitude, our focus should be on our own achievements rather than on figuring out what another person needs to reach that state.

D: Develop Your Environment

- Look around your house and place of work. In places of prominence (above the calendar, on the side of a mirror, on the desktop, etc.), place encouraging and uplifting quotations. Make up your own positive statements and add or exchange them for upbeat phrases or pictures.

- Keep supportive talk tapes and mind-strengthening tapes in the car to be reminded of the right and progressive perspective, and listen to them on the way to work and back home. Even uplifting and joyous music has a similar effect on our thinking. For those who are religiously inclined, an abundance of uplifting spiritual guidance material is available on books and tapes for review.

- Color and design your physical surroundings in light and bright colors, keeping them clean and clutter free. Use adequate lighting and use full-spectrum light (for example, Vita-Lite, Grow lux, etc.) to keep up spirits, especially in the winter months, when sunlight availability is diminished. Walks in the mall can be helpful for some of those dreary months.

Chapter 6

In a Nutshell

"The world is a looking glass, and gives back to every man the reflection of his own face."
~William Makepeace Thackery

The things we see are often reflections of our own thoughts and perceptions of a stimulus. If one is able to understand this, the situation, environment, and interaction will not matter anymore. Possibilities, opportunities, cheerfulness, and peace will abound.

Successful people in the real estate business often say that the most important thing when investing in property is "Location, location, and location!" Similarly, the most important ingredient in the recipe of successful life is attitude, attitude, and attitude!

Williams James appropriately said,

> *"Human beings, by changing the inner attitudes of their minds, can change the outer aspects of their lives."*

The way we feel, the way we react, the actions we take, and the emotions we generate are all functions of how we perceive situations. Once we realize this, it is within us to alter that perception and therefore alter our feelings, thoughts, and actions. Only a positive disposition can generate a positive outcome. And if we have the right attitude, even if we are incapable of changing our external circumstances, we can still feel content, peaceful, and in harmony.

To sum up the immense role of this single aspect of mind on the outcome of an individual, probably no one has said it better than Charles Swindoll:

"The longer I live, the more I realize the impact of attitude on life. Attitude, to me, is more important than facts. It is more important than the past, than education, than money, than circumstances, than failures, than success, than what other people think or say or do...we cannot change our past...we cannot change the inevitable. The only thing we can do is play on the one string we have, and that is our attitude... I am convinced that life is 10% what happens to me and 90% how I react to it. And so it is with you...we are in charge of our attitudes."

—Charles Swindoll

Progressive Thoughts and Habits

Chapter 7

Thoughts and Habits

"Change your thoughts and you change your world."
~Norman Vincent

Years ago, when Vincent made that statement, he had little knowledge that scientific advances would make that possible. Recently, neurosurgeons at New England Sinai Hospital in Massachusetts were able to implant a brain chip in a paralyzed patient; the chip helped to read his thoughts via computer.[2] By connecting these signals to motor devices, it has become possible to transform the patient's thoughts into motion. This ingenious work of Professor John Donoghue only goes to show the power of our thoughts.

The effects of our thought processes and the habits they generate have great impact on the lives that we lead. If you look around, you will notice three kinds of people. First, and most commonly, there are those who seem to be running from pillar to post, living a chaotic and inefficient life. These people appear confused most of the time, are poor achievers, and (of prime importance) are never at ease. Then there is a variety that does not get much accomplished but doesn't care about it anyway. Finally, there are those who seem to have everything under control, know what to do, and are peaceful and rested. These are the people who are most successful. It is natural to be drawn to them; they are popular, and most people seek their advice and company. If you are one of the lucky ones from the third category, you have already overcome one of the greatest hurdles in life.

---

[2] URL- http://news.bbc.co.uk/2/hi/health/4396387.stm

A healthy attitude allows the mind to be fertile in its conception of ideas and in the execution of proposals. The former is referred to as *progressive thoughts*, and the latter is referred to as *promotional habits*. If an individual has a sound combination of these two, he or she can achieve practically anything desired. And it is this fulfillment of internal needs, expectations of the self, and contentment with life that brings peace and tranquility to an individual. A remarkable analysis of movie stars showed that those who have achieved success and received awards or recognition for their work tend to live longer than those who have not. So what is it that makes some successful and others regretful? The answer is that the outcome in life is caused by two aspects of utmost importance: the thoughts and habits of an individual.

> *"We sow our thoughts, and we reap our actions.*
> *We sow our actions, and we reap our habits.*
> *We sow our habits and we reap our characters.*
> *We sow our characters, and we reap our destiny."*
> ~Anonymous

Chapter 8

What Are Progressive Thoughts?

"As you think, you travel, and as you love you attract. You are today where your thoughts have brought you; you will be tomorrow where your thoughts take you."
~James Lane Allen

Thoughts are ideas that invade or inhabit our minds, while habits are behaviors and actions that have become part of our lives. We all know how some thoughts and habits that we harbor help us achieve what we desire, but there are also some that actually hinder that process.

The power of thoughts and their impact on health has been evaluated in many clinical studies. In a study from Denmark published a few years ago, the researchers who looked at the effect of thoughts, including ruminations and feelings of sadness, on subjective sleep quality, immune system strength (as measured by cell counts and immune cell activity) and health care utilization concluded that *"negative thoughts may be detrimental to health, independently of negative affect."* [3]

Thoughts and habits that make it easier for us to attend to our responsibilities, work toward our goals, and help build positive character are bound to promote our well-being. But many of us,

---

[3] Thomsen, D.K., M. Y. Mehlsen, M. Hokland, A. Viidik, F. Olesen, K. Avlund, K. Munk, and R. Zachariae. Negative thoughts and health: associations among rumination, immunity, and health care utilization in a young and elderly sample. *Psychosomatic Medicine.* 2004 May–Jun. 66(3): 363-71

because of our busy and chaotic lives, have not had an opportunity to stop and think about what these are and how to enhance them. The analysis of these is the key to success in almost every winning situation.

The key elements of ideas and behaviors that promote success tend to be the following:

1. *Principle Driven:*

Each person needs to have a clear understanding of what is inherently important to him or her, as well as an order of importance of these items. For example, a mother may feel that attending to her dependent kids is her prime objective, while an executive of a firm may find that the promotion of his company is his major concern. There may be some who feel that both family and career need to be harmoniously successful for them to feel satisfied. In any of these situations, clarification and prioritization of these items is of prime importance. These are the fundamental principles that should guide our thoughts.

2. *Character Building:*

For any idea to have a lasting and positive impact on your life, it is essential that it be in harmony with the values that humanity promotes. Honest, courageous, compassionate, and loyal ideas that are conceived with long-term effects in mind are bound to bear fruit for eternity. Short-term, quick fixes with deceitful intentions are going to produce short-lived results that will end up harming the individual who employs them.

Ideas aimed at the mere acquisition of wealth are often less satisfying than what they may have appeared at the outset. In fact, an increase in wealth invariably leads to the desire for more and pushes an individual into a vicious cycle. In the words of Lucius Annaeus Seneca, a Roman author,

> *"Many a man has found the acquisition of wealth only a change, not an end, of miseries."*

On the other hand, ideas that promote development of character and thrive on the virtuous qualities of an individual have an amazingly long-lasting, satisfying quality. If you have ever helped an individual in distress, you know that feeling.

3. Simple and Goal Oriented:

The twenty-first century has brought with it glamour, superficial glitter, and pressures to acquire luxurious items to an extent that we have started forgetting our real needs—the needs to promote our inner-worth, develop values, and keep life simple; we need these things in order to truly experience inner well-being. Our thoughts have accordingly gotten so twisted, complicated, and layered that we are unable to recognize what thoughts would be satisfying. And yet, the most rewarding times for us are interactions with ourselves or a loved one. The world-renowned American physicist Albert Einstein said it very well:

> *"Possessions, outward success, publicity, luxury—to me these have always been contemptible. I assume that a simple and unassuming manner of life is best for everyone, best for both the body and the mind."*

While simplicity in thought and action helps an individual to conserve energy and allow mental faculties to be channeled in the appropriate direction, focus allows one to reach his or her goals with ease. The success of one of the most outstanding achievers in modern times, Bill Gates, may have many attributes. However, as he has pointed out, focus is an essential component of his success.

> *"My success, part of it certainly, is that I have focused in on a few things."*
>
> ~Bill Gates, Chairman of Microsoft

Chapter 9

How Do We Change Our Thoughts?

The first step, and probably the most important one, in changing our thoughts is realizing our shortcomings and putting in efforts to gain the wisdom for improvement. By reading the works of great minds and communicating with accomplished men and women, one can gain insight and have opportunities to observe successful strategies. Only great minds can support great ideas; this notion is reflected well in the words of a great author:

> *"Keep away from people who try to belittle your ambitions. Small people always do that, but the really great make you feel that you, too, can become great."*
> ~Mark Twain (Samuel L. Clemens)

The next step toward ensuring any change is to firmly incorporate this wisdom in our minds so that it influences our behavior and actions through a process called *learning*. Psychologists refer to learning as a process achieved through either conditioning or cognitive application. While the former refers to the use of rewards or punishments to reinforce changes in practice, the latter uses thinking and reasoning to the same effect. By utilizing both mechanisms and involving observation, insight, positive reinforcement, and reward, one can favorably influence the mental faculties to indulge in progressive thoughts.

Unfortunately, not all learned behavior stays with us forever unless efforts are made to retain it. This is where we need to pay special attention to optimizing our memory to retain such changes. Repeatedly reviewing and monitoring our thoughts can help us ensure prolonged benefits from this change in thinking.

We often forget that although our mind has limitless potential, it does need to concentrate and be focused on limited tasks for optimum output. I prefer to call the energy available at any given time to focus and reach my potentials my "pool of mental energy." Distracting, inconsequential, and unproductive thoughts are unlikely to be associated with any benefit and are more likely to lower our potential by encroaching on our mental energies. Through conscious and repeated endeavors, we should weed out these thoughts and allow our fertile mental grounds to bear productive fruit. Keeping a clear vision of what is important in the long run, keeping our thoughts focused around our personal mission, and building our mental strengths around our mission is the only way of bringing success to realization.

It is equally important to keep in mind that we should first strive for excellence, not perfection. By striving for excellence, we are trying to do our best without pressuring ourselves to be perfect. This way we can enjoy the process of self-evolution without adding the stress of meeting set standards. As a result, the process tends to be enticing, not compelling. Also keep in mind that we are constantly in a dynamic—not static—state of existence. Like nature and life, where changes are inevitable, a strong mind is able to attend to diversity and flux. Be like a palm tree in a storm—ready to bend and survive rather than be severed by the storm.

There is one aspect that is of paramount importance to practice and inculcate, and that is the wisdom imparted by a great saint.

"Do not dwell in the past, do not dream of the future,
concentrate the mind on the present moment."

~Buddha

Hence we can see that concentration has been considered an attribute and quality of utmost significance that allows an individual to be able to achieve and progress since times immemorial.

Chapter 10

Promotional Habits

---

*"I know of no more encouraging fact than the
unquestioned ability of a man to elevate his life by
conscious endeavor."*
~Henry David Thoreau

As mortal creatures on this earth, we are constantly engaging in activities to sustain our livelihood. When a particular activity or behavior is repeatedly performed and becomes embedded in our actions, it becomes a habit. For example, you probably have been brushing your teeth every morning after waking up for so long now that it has become a habit. There are probably other actions that you may indulge in that may not be productive and in fact may be counterproductive.

One such example is neglecting important tasks for so long that there is not enough time for preparation. The consequences of this are poor results and late arrivals, which on most occasions will cause you many inconveniences or even harm your reputation. Unfortunately, if you do not realize what habits you are harboring and what effects they are having on your life, you will never be able to rise above your present state of existence. This is age-old wisdom that was described best in the words of a saint:

"Habit, if not resisted, soon becomes a necessity."
~Saint Augustine

45

If habits are that important, then what should we incorporate within us to help us to develop healthy and promotional habits? In my opinion, the component that is probably most important is discipline. The three crucial and pertinent issues pertaining to self-discipline are prioritizing and planning, developing organizational skills, and staying determined and motivated.

1. *Priority and Planning*

> *"It is the first of all problems for a man to find out what kind of work he is to do in this universe."*
> ~Thomas Carlyle

If you have ever been involved in building a house, you realize how important it is to have a blueprint before you begin to build. Imagine doing it the other way around! Unless you know what to do and how to do it, it is almost impossible to do it!

The other aspect of planning is figuring out what your short-term plans and long-term plans are. It is probably better to have your long-term plans drawn out first, because they may alter your short-term options. If you have negotiated the first step of setting priorities, this will be easier. For example, say you eventually see yourself as a successful businessman. Then it will make more sense to take that not-so-enticing class on accounting instead of the interesting class on history, for as a Bavarian proverb goes:

> *"What is the use of running when we are on the wrong road?"*

But how do we know for sure where we should be headed? How should we figure out our destiny? How can we see the future? The answer is that we don't. No one can predict the future with certainty. One can only dream and work toward fulfilling those dreams. And most successful people will tell you that that is what they started with— just dreams. In the words of the famous Italian artist Michelangelo,

> *"Lord, grant that I may always desire more than I accomplish."*
> ~Michelangelo Buonarroti

Some pessimists will say, "Be realistic; not every dream is fulfilled." This may be true, but how will you ever know if you have never tried? And the labor will never be lost, for you will have enjoyed working toward what you really wanted. But I firmly believe that you can have what you want if you have the capability, commitment, and concentration to strive for your goal. I am reminded of the time when I had to revise five years' worth of studies in two months to be able to pass a test. Many previous students warned me that it was close to impossible and that I should wait for six months for the next exam date. I thought to myself, *Worst comes to worst, I will have to do just that, but why don't I at least try?* I worked hard and attended to my priority with true dedication. I cannot describe the feeling I felt when the results were released. I knew that I had just witnessed a fulfilled dream.

Ask any great athlete if he or she was born with his or her skills. Most athletes, if not all, will say that once they realized their capabilities and interests, they worked hard to achieve their goal. So look at yourself, talk to yourself, and find out for yourself where you are headed. The bottom line is that you should listen to everyone, but do what your mind tells you to.

> *"The world judge of men by their ability in their professions, and we judge ourselves by the same test; for it is on that on which our success in life depends."*
> ~William Hazlitt

Clearly, one needs to be realistic, too. Someone who is five feet tall and forty-eight years old is unlikely to ever play in the NBA. The next thing one needs to consider is where his talent lies or what he can learn that holds his interest. The famous German author Johan Wolfgang von Goethe phrased this especially well:

"The man who is born with a talent which he is meant to use finds his greatest happiness in using it."

While prioritizing helps us see *where* we are headed, planning is the understanding of *how* we are headed there. This can be illustrated in undertaking a journey. You may decide that you are headed to Chicago, but planning allows you to realize how it would be best for you to get there given the constraints on time and finances. Needless to say, planning is as important as prioritizing!

Two important resolutions can help you make great strides toward this objective. Firstly, starting today, sit down with yourself for some time and reflect on past and present experiences. Now visualize the future and observe which relationships, environments, and positions provide you with the most sense of comfort, joy, and peace. Those things should embody the principles that guide your efforts. Secondly, allocate some time every day during which you will sit down with yourself to evaluate the day's events and prepare for the future. Utilize this time every day to organize those priorities. One of the most amazing and multifaceted achievers of all times, Benjamin Franklin, had a rigidly disciplined routine with time set aside for reflection and analysis. Some suggestions for organization are given ahead.

2. Organization and Progress

"I never did anything worth doing by accident; nor did any
of my inventions come by accident; they came by work."
~Thomas Alva Edison

The modern times have brought with them endless chores with limited personal resources. Take life from, say, the eighteenth century. Most families at that time had only one earning member, usually the paternal unit. The mother was devoted to rearing the children and managing the house. The chores outside the house got the attention of the father. Household help from other family members and other individuals was easily available. In effect, there was not too much to do; there were enough people around, and chores were neatly divided. Now look at our lives today. If you were to list the number of tasks a two-parent, earning family has to undertake, it could give us all a headache. Add to it the fact that many families are either single parent or complicated in nature, and it would be gargantuan set-up according to the values of our ancestors a century ago!

It is impossible to separate our mental peace from our physical demands. One cannot feel content and happy in chaotic surroundings. Whether it is caused by spatial disorganization, constraints of time, or demands of professional and family events, it is not unusual for anyone to feel overwhelmed and confused.

How are we to have a clear mind if there are continuous clouds of never-ending chores, messy surroundings, and no available time? If there is one book I could recommend that you should read to organize your life better, it would have to be Stephanie Winston's *Best Organizing Tips*. It is as complete a guide as possible for any person who feels that this is a weak skill for them. Everything under the sun that a mortal may need to comfortably, efficiently, and successfully cross the sea of life is right there. Here are some of my own practices and thoughts on the subject:

Spatial Organization: Whether it is at home or your work place, strive to keep your surroundings clean and in order. Most minds can perform optimally with a clean and well-organized background. As an example, imagine driving at the time of day when traffic is at its most chaotic. You waste much more effort, energy, and time traveling the same distance than you would on an uncrowded road on a weekend. The same is true for the mind; it needs to have a clear space with references in the right places that are quick at hand to expedite the thought process. Firstly, create—and if needed, label—a space for all the essentials. Have you ever looked at those drawer organizers that have twenty or more slots that are pictorially labeled so that paper clips, tape, pens, and other objects can easily be organized in those spots? If you share a household with other family members, make sure each person is involved in the organization. Don't let the paperwork flood your life. Make quick decisions as to which papers need to be pitched, which need to be read at leisure, and which need to be filed. Having filing cabinets for personal, professional, and financial papers can go a long way toward conserving time and energy when retrieving information.

Time Management: There is an old Asian proverb that says, "Time doesn't care for those who do not care for it." One of the most useful seminars I attended was on managing time to get the most possible work done. Not only did this teach me to get my assignments done on time, plan my future projects appropriately, and attend to family demands, but it also allowed me to have extra time for personal leisure. Needless to say, the mental tranquility all this brought was priceless.

Essentially, time management has two main components: a work list prioritized by importance and deadlines, and a timetable. For the latter, it is recommended to use a calendar (pocket, wall, or desk) that has each month on a separate sheet with days displayed as boxes. From the work list, enter items in the boxes according to when they need to be attended to. Now divide each day into thirty-minute blocks. Put items from the work list in those slots depending on the time of the day, the location, or the intensity of the projects that need to be done. Allow yourself a few minutes of break between long stretches, but remember to keep them brief. You will be surprised at how much extra time there is in a day that we simply never realized was there because we were busy wasting it in meaningless activities. Electronic organizers and even cell phones have these functions with alarms to remind you what to do and when to do it!

In fact, it is easy to plan ahead for days and even months. Activities and events, if known in advance, can be placed on the calendar to help plan each day and also to serve as reminders for the future. Driving with precise directions can get you where you want; just sitting behind the wheel and grumbling will get you nowhere.

3. Determination and Motivation

"Courage and perseverance have a magical talisman, before which difficulties disappear and obstacles vanish into air."

~John Quincy Adams

Not uncommonly, we start a task with a lot of enthusiasm but with time lose our drive. It is only natural for a human to be lazy. Perhaps if we were still living in the Stone Age, it would have mattered little if we rested all day after hunting for one meal for the day. We would have no work to worry about, no schooling, no activities, and no CNN! But alas, thanks to some inquisitive and enthusiastic humans and their astonishing discoveries, we have much more complicated lives than our predecessors had—lives in which procrastination only brings failure, despair, and a vicious cycle of doom.

So here we are, as much in need for continued motivation as initial determination. Probably the most often-used learning strategy is to face the natural consequences. That can be extremely detrimental to future progress, and it can be difficult to reverse (as in the case of losing a desirable job due to poor performance). The next best thing may be to imagine the consequences. Or look at other people's negative experiences (or your own past dealings) to remind yourself of the possible negative consequences. Another useful technique is placing positive slogans around yourself (on the mirror, on your desk, etc.) and reading or listening to positive inspirational material.

Sometimes we do not realize the negative impact that people with negative attitudes have on us. What applies to another person may not apply to you. Circumstances, responsibilities, capabilities, and connections differ for each individual. You have to figure out for yourself what is the best course of action for you. On the other hand, getting an activity started in a group of well-meaning people may have its own rewards. Breaking down a difficult task over a period of time with rewards set up for yourself can be a fun way of handling a task. And if need be, getting help with a task so that you can conserve time and energy for more important things may help prevent fatigue and stress from taking away your drive.

Stress-free Mind

Chapter 11

Stressing over Stress

"No passion so effectively robs the mind of its powers of acting and reasoning as fear."

~Edmund Burke

The medical discovery that the greatest psychological contributor to ill health tends to be the presence of mental stress in an individual's life is extremely valuable. Whether or not this stress is related to fears in the professional, financial, personal, or social realms, it seems to have a significant negative influence on our feelings of comfort, balance, and harmony. Over a prolonged period, it is usually associated with medical problems, such as hypertension, heart attacks, anxiety, and depression. In fact, there is evidence to support the idea that it even alters our immune systems and thereby predisposes us to infections and maybe even cancers.

It is scientifically proven that there are serious psychological changes and life impairments in a condition called PSTD (post traumatic stress disorder).[4] This condition was first recognized after the Vietnam War when about 15 percent of veterans were noted to have prolonged symptoms that negatively affecting their mental and physical health following completion of the war.

Real or perceived fears and the resulting stresses act in yet another way to lower potential and well-being. Fear acts as a deterrent to

---

[4] URL- http://www.ncptsd.va.gov/ncmain/ncdocs/fact_shts/fs_what_is_ptsd.html

constructive and imaginative thinking, lowers creativity, and hence decreases the chances of finding solutions to problems. The result is the persistence of problems or a worsening of the situation, both of which compound fear and stress. This causes the vicious cycle of fear, poor thinking, lack of solutions, poor outcome, and additional negative life situations, which causes feelings of fear, and thereby stress, to escalate.

Not uncommonly, parents repeatedly use fear to produce what they perceive as desirable results in their offspring. Although they may be happy to see immediate results, such repeated attempts are only going to reduce the mental creativity of their children. Repeated and prolonged fear essentially lowers a children's self-esteem, robs them of self-confidence, and takes away from them their trust. Like creepers without support, they are unable to reach the heights that they deserve to attain. "Where the mind is without fear, the head is held high!" (Rabindranath Tagore). Simple yet powerful, these words of a famous poet bring to our attention how uplifting it is to be stress free. Freedom from fear is indeed an essential prerequisite to mental health.

But clearly it is easy to say, "Try being without stress." It is like telling someone, "Don't have fever!" If it were within our power not to have fever or stress, who would not avoid those menaces? For a physician, it may be easy to give some helpful advice to avoid fever. Suggestions like avoiding crowded areas, washing hands before eating, taking plenty of fluids, taking appropriate medications, etc., are probably helpful in preventing and treating infective fevers. Similarly, there are simple yet helpful strategies that one can adopt in avoiding or managing our fears and stresses. Let us discuss some of them.

Chapter 12

Addressing and Managing Stress

In order to manage the stress that we encounter in our daily lives, we must first understand where this stress originates. The mind is a double-edged sword. On one hand it gives us thoughts that are necessary for our progress and productivity. On the other hand it can play havoc in our bodies by promoting feelings, emotions, and physiological reactions that make us uneasy and disturbed. This is often not because of any immediate, real threat, but because of a perpetuation of negative thought processes by the mind that often arise when we are not fully conscious of our mental state. These processes may cause the mind to perceive an erroneous sense of threat to survival. When this happens, the individual is locked in a state of negative energy with the accompanying physiological symptoms of tense muscles, increased heart rate, elevated blood pressure, and sometimes even labored breathing.

If one forces that very mind to completely concentrate on a physical object, an activity (breathing being the easiest), or a pleasant thought, the negative feeling, or stress, disappears. Similarly, using meditative techniques, you can rise, in your consciousness, above the realm of the disturbed mind. If you are able to enter a state of deep meditation in which you find a connection with the soul and are able to bring that experience back into waking consciousness, the effect is eternal. Saints and yogis who practice meditation on a regular basis are living examples of this blissful state. While we strive for that state, some simple measures may provide benefit in the meantime.

Attitude, Attitude, Attitude

"He that is discontented in one place will seldom be content in another."

~Aesop

Not too long ago, two families I know were anticipating moving to another state. It was amazing how different their approaches and perceptions of the events were, and the resultant mental and physical manifestations were obvious. One family was excited about the change. They viewed it as an opportunity to explore new surroundings, meet with challenges at the workplace, redo their rooms in a new house, make new friends, etc. They were exuding energy and enthusiasm. Members of the other family, on the other hand, were apprehensive, anxious and sad, and they seemed to be constantly voicing negative feelings. The apprehension and depression clearly did not serve them well. If anything, it slowed them further, diminished their interactive and adaptive skills, and diminished their vision. This much difference in outcome was caused just by a difference of attitude!

It is important to keep in mind that life is about living and enjoying the present. No wonder it is said: *"Yesterday is history, Tomorrow is a mystery. Today is a gift: that is why they call it the present."* Accept that everything is there for a reason; our narrow vision often prevents us from seeing this. Keeping a broadminded approach, finding opportunities in every situation, and attending to things proactively all help in maintaining the right perspective.

So before we blame our surroundings, grumble about other people, and make others and ourselves miserable, it is crucial to get an attitude check. (See the section on attitude for more.)

Our Social Surroundings

"Every man becomes, to a certain degree, what the people he generally converses with are."
~Philip Dormer Stanhope

Man is a social animal. He seeks the company of other humans, and he is fairly easily influenced by them. This is especially so for those of us who have not set out for ourselves a core set of values and vision. On the other hand, those who have mastered their minds with positive strengths often serve to influence others in a productive manner. Therefore, until we find ourselves in that desirable state, it is to our benefit to keep the company of individuals who share their positive mental strength. You may call it social mentoring; it is never too late to learn from others.

Probably the most effective way of recognizing such individuals is by simple observations without personal involvement. The next time you are in a social gathering or in the company of another person, closely observe their behavior, their choices of words, and their emotional reactions. Notice if these are repeated patterns, and note whether the environment this individual provides is uplifting or depressive. Make notes based on these observations as to whether you should increase or diminish your interactions with this person. The people you do this with may be relatives, friends, social acquaintances, colleagues at work, or even neighbors. In fact, the most desirable achievement in this realm is finding a soul mate—one who listens, gives advice when asked, is never derogatory, sees and explains all perspectives, and maintains a sense of humor, honor, and dignity.

Sometimes we may indulge in passive interactions that can have significant influences on our thought processes if we are not careful. A few years ago, I noticed in my reflective hour for the day that my behavior toward others was showing elements of criticism and anger, which I usually condemn. In fact, I was developing an argumentative temperament that was only acting to my disadvantage. I subsequently started examining my daily interactions and influences more carefully. Interestingly, I realized that I had started listening to a radio talk show aired by an extremely biased, opinionated, and aggressive speaker. He seemed to be continuously harping on the negative words, behaviors, and actions of socially recognized people. Due to my job responsibilities during that time, I was spending more than two hours in the car per day while invariably listening to this spicy talk. I observed how angry and upset I felt about issues that were beyond my immediate concern and that I had no way of influencing! Sometimes I could even feel my jaw and fist tightening due to the provocative talk. Little had I realized that this influence was slowly corroding the very principles that I had strived to adopt. I had started to become all the things I disliked in others. Needless to say, that was the last day I ever tuned in to that radio channel!

One other aspect that we sometimes ignore though it can have a significant effect on our personal and social bearing is our communication skills. The tone of conversation and the choice of words we use can alter another person's perception of the matter despite our best intentions guiding our actions. Conversing with empathy, understanding, patience, and open-mindedness prevents unnecessary stresses in relationships.

Anticipating Periods of Stress

Chemicals called hormones continuously bathe our internal organs. These can alter our sense of perception or make us more anxious than what our circumstances dictate. An example is an individual who has witnessed a life-threatening event. His or her body has had an outpouring of chemicals like cortisol and epinephrine. These make the individual restless and anxious, and they put him or her in a state of anticipating the worst. In women there are monthly cyclical changes in hormones that are known to make them irritable and over-reactive in addition to feeling restless and moody. Paying special attention to the mind's and body's needs at these times can be very helpful in preventing full-blown crisis situations. Making a special note of a diet that gives a sense of peace and ease can serve an important function in such anticipated times of stress.

Chapter 13

Time for Mental Tranquility

Our minds are constantly functioning; even during sleep there are neurochemical events and synaptic electric activity occurring. It is like an engine that is continuously running. Whether good or bad, thoughts are constantly running through this amazing organ. How can we provide it with the rest that it needs even in an awake state? The most effective way is engaging in meditation.

Meditation

Meditation has been used for many years, and it has even been studied for its beneficial effect on physiological and psychological states in humans. It is essentially a simple yet extremely powerful way to release and recharge the mental system with positive energy. As little as fifteen minutes of meditation a day is enough to have a significant positive influence on the psyche of an individual.

Scientifically, brain wave analyses of individuals during meditation have shown high alpha wave activity (slower and deeper waves than normal awake-state beta waves) in comparison to non-meditative groups, thereby confirming the relaxing effect of this experience. [5] Using breathing techniques combined with concentrative mental Qi Gong technique, researchers in China have observed even deeper

---

[5] Khare, K. C. and S. K. Nigam. A study of electroencephalogram in meditators. *Indian J Physiology & Pharmacology.* 2000 Apr; 44(2): 173-8

and slower theta brain waves, which occur during the stage of mental tranquility just before deep sleep is reached.

Extensive literature is available on this subject, and the reader is encouraged to read more; in the meantime, let me acquaint you with what I learned more than twenty years ago in my medical school, which I still consider a powerful meditation method.

Two simple ways of transcending the body and mind may be used to reach a state of relaxation, peace, refreshment, and rejuvenation. When you are least rushed, select a quiet area where you are unlikely to be disturbed. Sit in a relaxed position. (Sitting cross-legged, or Indian style, called *Sukhasan* in Yoga postures, is recommended, but not essential.) In case you have limited time, it is acceptable to use a timer so that you do not have to worry about looking at a watch or clock repeatedly. Create a word that has no meaning. (This is often termed *mantra*, meaning the mental tool that serves as a mystical, magical key and is usually given by a spiritual leader.) Close your eyes and start reciting it in your mind. In case thoughts come to your mind, let them pass without reacting to them. You will reach a state in which there are no thoughts in the mind; this is often accompanied by a feeling of complete relaxation. It may take a number of sessions to reach this state; persistence and practice will help you to eventually reach this blissful state of mental tranquility. Prolong this period as long as possible, and then gradually re-enter the material world. This period of gap in your thoughts is where you find the peace that your mind hides from you by creating a veil of constant thought.

On similar lines, an effective and traditional yogic meditation involves transcending the layers of the body by visualizing. In this form of meditation, sit in a quiet place in a relaxed posture. In case sitting is physically difficult, you may lie on your back with your arms a few inches from the sides of your body and your legs straight with a few inches of distance between the feet. This is called *Shavasan* (like the body of a lifeless person). Starting from the feet and moving toward the head, slowly clench and release, one by one, each muscle of the body. This is intended to penetrate the outer body layer. Thereafter, take a few deep breaths to enter the inner body. Using the vibrations of the word *Aum* three times, synchronize the internal milieu. Let thoughts be released from the mind with the calm belief that higher energy is taking care of any problems. Thereafter, relax in a thoughtless state and feel the inner soul. Visualize it connecting with the universal power, and draw energy and light into your spirit.

Another form of mental exercise performed and recommended by some to achieve positive results is referred to as *imagery*. This is somewhat similar to meditation, but it involves visualizing physical, mental, or social achievements desired by the individual. It has reportedly been used with success in some cases of cancer, where the affected person imagines the diminution of the tumor or cancer cells.[6]

In essence, all of these mind-relaxing techniques are geared toward creating a peaceful, refreshed, and sharp mental state. Many tapes, programs, and books are available to help individuals progress in their quests for mental tranquility by using the simple method of meditation.

---

[6] *Love, Medicine and Miracles* by Bernie S. Siegel, M.D.

Chapter 14

Other Ways of Addressing Stress

Life may be complicated, but it is essential that we make room in it for some fundamental stress relievers on a regular basis. Some of these are as follows.

1. Vacations

A simple and commonly employed method of mental rest is vacationing. It is important, however, not to take any work along during a vacation. Permitting the mind to completely decompress allows it to rejuvenate so that it can function more clearly upon returning to work. In my opinion, the words *vacation* and *work* just do not sound right together (vacate means to empty out). And in case you are planning to visit or stay with relatives during a vacation, make sure that you enjoy their company!

2. Music

Another form of uplifting experience comes from listening to rich music. In fact, music is one of the few arts that touch both the mind and spirits. Actively or passively enjoying the works of great artists such as Mozart, Bach, or Beethoven can soothe a disturbed mind beyond imagination, for as said Joseph Addison said:

> "Music, the greatest good that mortals know,
> And all of heaven we have below."

3. Humor

Similarly, funny and engrossing movies can serve as an excellent source of relaxation for the mind. Humor in any form is a well-known health promoter, and recent studies have confirmed that it boosts the immune system and lowers the recurrence of heart attacks. The age-old saying "Laughter is the best medicine" is not without merit.

4. Reading

Undoubtedly, the easiest and most mind-refreshing forms of entertainment to carry around are good books. There is no easier way of communicating with great minds and rejuvenating your own mind than by reading books. Even great minds feel that way, as is made evident by the words of a famous French author:

> "When I am attacked by gloomy thoughts nothing helps me so much as running to my books. They absorb me quickly and banish the clouds from my mind."
> ~Michel Eyquem de Montaigne

Body Over Mind?

There are indeed some time-tested methods of relaxing the mind by using physical measures. One of the more popular ones is still widely used in the modern world: body massage. Using soothing herbal oils with natural aromatic properties with this technique has become very popular. It has also been shown to promote the release of certain growth hormones that have compositions similar to substances with anti-aging properties. Similarly, using aromatic candles allows the fragrance of soothing herbs to tranquilize the agitated mind (but beware of imported ones with excessive lead content).

You may have repeatedly heard that one should have a glass of cold water when one feels angry. Water is indeed the main constituent of the body, and it is a useful solute for waste excretion. Because of this, it should be little wonder that water, both internally and externally, could serve as a valuable companion. According to Ayurvedic sciences, certain food types, such as spicy and sour, tend to stimulate our mental faculties. On the other hand, milk-containing foods (especially yogurt) and sweet items are soothing to our mind.

Realization of the cyclical changes that occur internally, including hormonal fluctuations and other cycles with mental influences (such as the menstrual cycle in women) is important. Doing so helps us to prepare and take measures to amend the consequences. (Calcium, green tea, and yogurt can be beneficial.) Similarly, the external influences of weather changes can be counteracted by appropriate measures.

Staying comfortably dressed, wearing the right kind of footwear, and maintaining a comfortable environmental temperature at home and at work can work wonders by helping you to avoid unnecessary physical stress and mental aggravation.

Chapter 15

Avoiding Stress

It is only fair to conclude that avoiding stress is as important as relieving stress. Staying away from situations that lower your well-being potential is an important method of preventing a downward spiral. Also, keeping in mind the ripple effect such situations have on our mental bearings should prompt us to catch ourselves early when we start perceiving such feelings. Allowing yourself some time each day to reflect on your thoughts, behavior, emotions, and actions is a highly recommended method. In case thoughts recur, especially during bedtime, writing them down and reflecting on them and then acting on them with a fresh mind can be much more productive. In fact, just the process of writing disturbing thoughts down helps lower the intensity of negative feelings and provides breathing space for more progressive thoughts.

Additionally, constant reminders in the form of motivational slogans, the realization that more harm than good is the net result of constant fear, and the understanding of physical and mental deterioration from stress and panic can all serve as deterrents to promoting a depressive state.

Needless to say, staying organized and disciplined and choosing the right companions and work environment can cause profound improvements to our health. In fact, according to some studies, work-related stresses are the prime psychological factor contributing to cardiovascular diseases in adults. In addition, paying close attention to our communication skills while maintaining clear and sincere intentions can ensure healthy and joyful relationships. If we keep in mind the simple truth stated below, a peaceful mind and blissful soul will be a reality:

> *"There is only one way to happiness, and that is to cease worrying about things which are beyond the power of our will."*
>
> ~Epictetus

Body

"Grace is to the body what clear thinking is to the mind."
~Francois de La Rochefoucauld

We all have a physical form that helps us manifest ourselves to others in addition to serving many other functions. We expect a lot from our bodies: to take us places, to do all kinds of chores, to play sports, to engage in various forms of physical activities, etc. And yet how much do we know about it? How well do we treat it? Do we provide it what it needs to keep it healthy? If not, then it is about time we paid it its dues. Learn about it, understand its needs, respect its diversity, provide the essentials, and protect it from the adverse.

While our mental health and spiritual health also have far-reaching influences on our physical state, there are three simple aspects that, if attended to with sincerity, can optimize our physical dynamism. Attention to these aspects is required for healthy existence and is therefore discussed in detail as:

- Vital Nutrition

- Energizing Activity

- Rejuvenating Rest

Vital Nutrition

Chapter 16

The Physical Body

"One's eyes are what one is, one's mouth what one becomes."

~John Galsworthy

What goes into that mouth of ours serves as the building blocks for our body. Each cell, each tissue, and each organ in our body is continuously renewed; we have a dynamic state of existence, which is the very reason we are alive. Just like what you feed and treat a plant with is going to determine its state, the body responds to what you put into it. An interesting experiment conducted on twins with healthy natural food versus junk food showed improved psychosocial and memory performance in the child receiving wholesome food.[7]

Food may affect not only our structures, but also our minds. To further our understanding of this simplified process, let us look at what the body is all about.

Body Structure

"Body says what the words cannot."

~Martha Graham

---

[7] URL- http://news.bbc.co.uk/2/low/health/2984519.stm

The body of a healthy adult male on an average is physically composed of the following main elements: protein (about 18 percent), fat (15 percent), and water (60 percent). All of these compounds, at an atomic level, are essentially some combination of C (carbon), H (hydrogen), O (oxygen), and N (nitrogen). In addition, there are many minor elements (vitamins) and minerals (7 percent) that constitute the body.[8] Women tend to have a higher percentage of fat than men, and the body's composition also changes somewhat with age. These constituents are arranged in cells, which form tissues, which in turn form organs. Organs with similar functions form systems, such as the skeletal system, the cardiovascular system, the muscular system, etc.

Body Fat Percentage Categories

The percentage of fat in our body varies with the gender and the athletic predisposition of an individual. The body fat designated as essential is lower than the recommended fat composition of a healthy body. This has been delineated as follows by the American Council of Exercise (ACE).*

*American Council on Exercise

Classification	Women (% fat)	Men (% fat)
Essential Fat	10-12%	2-4%
Athletes	14-20%	6-13%
Fitness	21-24%	14-17%
Acceptable	25-31%	18-25%
Obese	32% plus	25% plus

---

[8] *Review of Medical Physiology* by William Ganong

Complex chemical processes that occur in the body, called *metabolic pathways*, involve fats, proteins, and carbohydrates. While the body is capable of synthesizing different substances, there are certain fatty acids and amino acids that are needed by the body because they cannot be synthesized by it. These are called essential fatty acids and amino acids. The deficiency of these products can have negative structural and functional consequences. Therefore, it is not a good idea to live only on protein or only on fat. An adult body needs approximately 0.8 grams per kilogram per day of protein, which amounts to about fifty-six grams for a healthy, average-sized young man and approximately forty-five grams per day for a woman. These needs are not stationary; a change in body physiology changes the needs. For example, in pregnancy, when fetal tissue is being rapidly laid down, and because of the growing need of supporting organs in a woman's body, this need increases by an additional thirty grams per day to a total of seventy grams per day! Similarly, during illnesses with need for repair, higher protein intake is desirable.

Food: The Building Blocks

The food that we eat is essentially a combination of protein, fat, or carbohydrates as major molecules. Food provides calories that can be converted into energy needed for all kind of body activities. The amount of energy that can be released from a food product is dependent on its composition. Fat provides the most calories per gram (9.3 kcal/g) in comparison to carbohydrates and protein (approximately 4 kcal/g). These calories, if not consumed, are stored as fat in the body. Food also serves as the building blocks for our body. Fats, when broken down, furnish fatty acids, while proteins form amino acids. Carbohydrates are broken down into simple sugars, which circulate in the blood or get stored in the liver as complex sugars.

After extensive research, the U.S. Department of Health and Human Service recommends a certain combination of food products to serve as a balanced diet, and with good reason. They suggested the pyramid model to show that there should be a large intake of grain, vegetables, and fruits. The narrow tip, however, depicts the very small amount of fat and sweets that should be consumed. More recently, the food pyramid has been modified as a three-dimensional picture symbolizing personalization, gradual improvement, physical activity, variety, and moderation of different food categories.[9]

Therefore, in meal composition, paying close attention to include the following items throughout the day would go a long way toward attaining and maintaining good physical health:

- Three ounces of whole grain cereal/bread/rice/pasta

- Plenty of dark green, orange, and other vegetables

- Variety of fruits—fresh, frozen, or dried

- *Low fat milk/milk products, or a calcium-rich diet if lactose intolerant

- *Low-fat meat or poultry, beans, peas, nuts, and seeds

- Minimal intake of sweets or fatty foods, such as desserts and butter

(* Recently, concerns with the use of chemicals including hormones and pesticide, especially in dairy and meat products, have prompted the use of organic products)

This should roughly provide the needed calories, proteins, and essential elements of your body. An estimate of the serving size can be acquired by keeping the serving size within the size of your palm. Again, keeping on the low side where fat is concerned, drinking plenty of water, and keeping physically active will help you maintain

---

[9] URL- http://www.mypyramid.gov/

a healthy weight. Keep in mind the importance of eliminating hidden and unnecessary calories and fat. For example, eating salads is great, but it's no good if your dressing has fourteen grams of fat in a tablespoon! Eggs are excellent sources of complete protein and should be an integral part of a healthy diet as long as their yolks (rich in cholesterol) are not consumed with the same zest as their whites! Following is a listing of some common food items and their compositions so that you can recognize what you are ingesting.

Food composition

Food Product	Calories*	Fat*	Protein*
Grains			
Regular bread 1 slice	50-70	1g	2g
Fat-free bread 1 slice	35	0g	2g
Rice (cooked) 1 cup	160	1g	4g
White flour tortilla 1 medium	120	2g	2g
Wheat tortilla 1 medium	110	2g	2g
Vegetables			
Carrots ½ cup	30	0.1g	0.7g
Peas ½ cup	60	0.4g	4g
Spinach ½ cup	30	0.5g	0.5g
Corn ½ cup	60	0.6g	2g
Asparagus ½ cup	20	0.1g	1g
Green beans ½ cup	20	0g	1g
Fruits			
Banana 1 medium	100	0.4g	0.8g
Apple 1 medium	80	0.5g	0.3g
Orange ½ cup	60	0.3g	0.8g
Pineapple ½ cup	40	0.6g	0.4g
Peaches ½ cup	50	0g	0.6g
Milk & Products			
4% Milk 1 cup	150	9g	8g
Skim milk 1 cup	80	0g	8g
Yogurt 1 cup	150-200	8-9g	6-9g
Fat-free yogurt 1 cup	85-120	0g	7-12g
Cheese 1 slice	60	5g	3-5g
Fat-free cheese 1 slice	35-40	0g	3-5g
Cream cheese 1oz	70	5g	4g
Fat-free cream cheese 1 oz	30	0g	4g

Meat & Eggs

1 egg (white & yolk)	70	4g	6g
1 egg (white only)	25	0g	6g
Bologna 1 slice	60-70	4g	2g
Bacon 1 slice	60-70	5g	2g
Tuna (light) (1/4 cup)	60	1g	13g
Turkey 4 thin slices	60	2g	11g
Chicken breast 3 oz	120	3g	21g
Shrimp 3 oz	60	0g	13g

Legumes

Kidney beans ½ cup	110	1g	7g
Soy beans ½ cup	120	1g	12g
Garbanzo beans ½ cup	100	1g	6g
Pinto beans ½ cup	110	1g	7g
Lima beans ½ cup	115	0.5g	6g
Tofu 3 oz	45	1g	6g

Sugar, Fat & Nuts

Butter 1 tbsp	100	11g	0g
Chips 1 oz	150	10g	2g
Chocolate	170	10g	3g
Oreo cookie, 2	120	10g	2g
Peanuts 1 oz	160	14g	8g
Cashews 1 oz	170	14g	5g
Pistachios 1 oz	160	13g	6g

Some variations may occur depending on processing, serving size, sweetness, etc.

Chapter 16

Some Special Food Products

It would be an oversight not to mention some of the amazing health benefits that selected food products offer. Although the list here is not complete, there are certain food products that deserve special mention because of their constitution. Inclusion of these in our diet, even in small quantities, can be beneficial. However, it is prudent to mention that not all mentioned benefits have been scientifically proven by clinical studies. Some of these selected foods include the following:

1. **Yogurt**
2. **Broccoli, Tomatoes & Carrots**
3. **Banana, Berries & Apples**
4. **Fish**
5. **Nuts**
6. **Soy**
7. **Tea**
8. **Honey**
9. **Spinach**

These items are discussed below, and references are provided for more details as footnotes and in the suggested reading list.

Yogurt[10]

Probably one of the most amazing discoveries in food products has been the realization of the benefit of yogurt. Yogurt is a culture

---

[10] URL- http://www.csa.com/discoveryguides/probiotic/review4.php

of "friendly" bacteria called probiotics. These offer a multitude of benefits to the gut by improving intestinal immune response and digestibility, possibly reducing allergies, and adding important vitamins to our diet. At least one serving a day of unsweetened yogurt is definitely recommended.

Broccoli, Tomatoes & Carrots[11, 12]

Antioxidants in the form of phytochemicals found in vegetables like tomatoes (lycopene), broccoli (sulforaphane glucosinolate), and carrots (carrotenoids) are considered to be anti-aging and maybe even anti-cancer elements. Garlic, which is added as a spice to meals, provides a phytochemical called allicin. These antioxidants prevent damage to body cells by free radicals that form as a result of cell breakdown within the body.

Bananas, Berries & Apples[13-16]

The banana is an amazing fruit. It is rich with minerals such as iron, magnesium, and potassium, which may have a lowering effect on blood pressure. In addition, its fiber content helps regulate bowel activity and enhances intestinal health. It can also serve as an excellent source of instant energy due to its glucose, sucrose, and fructose concentrations. Berries, with their lycopene constituent, offer a vital antioxidant to the body that aids against aging and inflammation. Acai berries (grown in Central and South America) and Goji berries (grown in Tibet, the Himalayas, and Mongolia, also known as

---

[11] URL- http://news.bbc.co.uk/2/hi/health/4688854.stm
[12] URL- http://www.hsph.harvard.edu/nutritionsource/fruits.html
[13] URL- http://whfoods.org/genpage.php?tname=foodspice&dbid=7
[14] URL- http://news.bbc.co.uk/1/hi/health/4632886.stm
[15] URL- http://news.bbc.co.uk/2/hi/uk_news/magazine/5315202.stm
[16] URL- http://www.applepolyphenols.com/studies/cornell.htm

wolfberries and available in dried form in stores), are extremely rich in minerals, vitamins, and antioxidants.

Antioxidant contents are often measured by ORAC units (Oxygen Radical Absorbance Capacity) and help protect cells against oxidative damage. These have been shown to slow aging in rats by improving memory and performance of the nervous system and by protecting blood capillaries from damage. Other benefits, such as the prevention of cancer, have been attributed to fruits and vegetables with high ORAC units. (Spices, such as clove, turmeric, and cinnamon and cocoa also have high ORAC units).

The benefits of apples, which are promoted by the saying, "An apple a day keeps the doctor away," have been supported in health news. This has followed the detection of anti-cancer, anti-inflammatory, and antiviral activity in the extracts of apple, possibly due to chemicals such as flavonoids, polyphenols, and vitamin C. It is important to keep in mind that some of these substances are found only in the peel of the fruit.

Grapes, rich in antioxidants due to the presence of phytochemicals (e.g. resveratrol, which has been popular in the health industry due to claims of protection against cancer, promotion of brain and heart health, and anti-aging properties), have also been shown to release nitric oxide in the cells lining the blood vessels, and they may help prevent high blood pressure and heart problems.[17]

Fish[18,19]

Omega fatty acid found in certain fishes (opt for ocean or wild-catch fish rather than farm-grown fish to avoid mercury and other

---

[17] URL- http://www.ars.usda.gov/is/pr/1997/971120.htm
[18] URL- http://www.hsph.harvard.edu/press/releases/press10172006.html
[19] URL- http://www.epa.gov/mercury/advisories.htm

industrial wastes, such as PCBs) helps provide cardiovascular and nerve protection benefits. Six to twelve ounces of fish a week is considered enough to provide this benefit. For individuals who follow vegetarian diets, a once-a-week omega fatty acid supplement in capsule form may serve as a replacement. Walnuts also contain omega fatty acids, and small amounts of them may be used instead.

Nuts[20]

Among nuts, walnuts have some very beneficial properties that are worth discussing. They have been shown to be rich in arginine, antioxidants, alpha-linolenic acid, and omega-3 fatty acids. These constituents help the heart blood vessels maintain flexibility and might prevent fat deposits in the hearts blood vessels, which may lower the incidence of heart diseases.

Soy[21]

Soy has been considered a useful food product to keep handy due to its very high protein content and low carbohydrate and fat load. It has been shown to contain phytochemicals called isoflavones that lower LDL (low-density lipoprotein) and thus may aid in lowering the risk of heart attacks. Its high fiber and calcium content provide unique benefits in regulating bowel function and preventing osteoporosis. It also has phytoestrogen, which may be beneficial in eliminating hot flashes in postmenopausal syndrome and during the premenstrual period.

However, there have been some concerns raised about possible harmful health effects from soy products. It has protein enzyme

---

[20] URL- http://news.bbc.co.uk/2/hi/health/6036409.stm
[21] URL- http://www.ahrq.gov/clinic/epcsums/soysum.htm

inhibitors, which may affect digestion. In male rats, it decreased brain neurotrophic factors, which could result in dementia with prolonged and excessive intake. Also, probable contamination with aluminum and MSG during processing has raised concerns. Additionally, the absorption of some minerals may be hindered by soy products due to the high phytate concentration in soy, which in particular may affect thyroid gland function. Due to these considerations, it may be useful to avoid excess soy and to consider other good protein sources, such as egg whites and whey protein, especially for men.

Tea[22]

Tea has recently gained immense popularity for its content of polyphenolic compounds such as flavonoids and catechins, which are antioxidants and probably offer benefit against cancer and heart diseases. This may be more so in green tea than the oft-consumed black tea. In addition, tea has small amounts of certain valuable vitamins and minerals such as zinc, manganese, and potassium.

Honey[23]

Eating fresh fruits and vegetables is undoubtedly beneficial, but the benefits may be lost if juices laden with refined sugar are ingested instead. Honey is a unique natural sweetener with the goodness of antioxidants in addition to antibacterial effects. It may be a better substitute to refined sugar, and has been used extensively in traditional medicine for its therapeutic effects. However, keep in mind that excess of anything is harmful, and that honey is not recommended for those at risk of developing diabetes.

---

[22] URL- http://www.bbc.co.uk/health/healthy_living/nutrition/drinks_caff.shtml#tea
[23] URL- http://www.whfoods.org/genpage.php?tname=foodspice&dbid=96

Spinach[24]

Spinach* is yet another pro-health food product that is much discussed in health reviews. In addition to having anti-oxidants (methylenedioxyflavonol glucuronides and neoxanthin), it is a rich source of vitamins and minerals and is believed to promote health of the cardiovascular, gastrointestinal, and nervous systems. Being compulsive about thoroughly washing the vegetables could prevent exposure to biological and chemical toxins. (*There was an E. coli warning in some contaminated spinach sold in the recent past.)

[Another green plant causing a buzz in the health industry is Wheatgrass.[25] It was during a recent social gathering that I learned about the amazing recovery of the mother of one of my friends from advanced-stage lymphoma at the age of eighty with the daily use of wheatgrass. She had apparently been told that she would probably not live for longer than six months, and medications had been stopped, as the cancer was perceived to be terminal. For three years, however, she enjoyed remission! Wheatgrass has been reported to contain some very useful constituents for health benefits[25] including vitamins (vitamin E as alpha tocopherol succinate, vitamin B12, vitamin K, and folate) in addition to minerals like magnesium, iron, and potassium. The high content of chlorophyll contained in this product is claimed to provide immense energy and healing powers. Also, it is believed to contain large amounts of superoxide dismutase, a powerful antioxidant. However, wheatgrass is currently considered an alternative therapeutic supplement rather than a mainstream food product, and more scientific information is needed before the USDA[26] endorses it as a food product with health benefits. Make sure you read the precautions, such as higher risk of clot formation in predisposed individuals due to high vitamin K content, before jumping on the bandwagon.]

---

[24] Caldwell, C. R. Oxygen radical absorbance capacity of the phenolic compounds in plant extracts fractionated by high-performance liquid chromatography. *Analytic Biochemistry.* 2001 Jun 15; 293(2): 232-8.
[25] Wheatgrass: Nature's Finest Medicine By Steve Merowitz
[26] URL- http://plants.usda.gov/java/profile?symbol=PASM

Chapter 17

Water and Oil

Considering that 60 percent of the adult body is water and we are constantly cycling this fluid throughout the body, it is little wonder that it needs utmost attention. We lose water in our urine, stools, sweat, etc. All our waste products that need to be flushed by our kidneys are dependent on the availability of water as a solvent. Adults need a minimum of six to eight glasses to meet their daily needs. In addition, taken before meals, it lowers the stomach's capacity for food. The first thing we should put in our body is one to two glasses of water. Excessive amounts of plain water taken at one time when one is not thirsty can be dangerous due to its effects of hyponatremia (low sodium in the blood) and hypoosmolality (low tonicity of the blood), which can impair brain function. Occasionally adding a few drops of honey and lemon juice to a glass of water can offer further health benefits.

Interestingly, it is speculated by some that one of the reasons that weight becomes an issue with aging may be related to loss of thirst sensation with age. With the loss of thirst, one is more likely to have more food instead of having the water that is needed. The resultant chronic dehydration is detrimental to health. To ensure constant vigilance regarding this essential need, try to keep a daily water count. Alternatively, you can use the following system, which has worked well for me, after ensuring that you do not have any medical conditions related to kidney, heart or hormonal disorder to prevent adequate fluid intake:

Water glass first thing in the morning   2
Water glass before every meal   1 X 3
Water glass before and after exercising   1 X 2
Water glass after the last meal of the day   1

Since we are going to consume so much water, the question of prime importance is: Is it safe water? Water can contain both chemicals and organisms unless specifically treated. There are various forms of water treatment including chemical, filtration, osmosis, ultraviolet, ozone, etc. Many people use bottled water nowadays, which may be the product of springs, glaciers, wells, or even purified municipal water sources. It may, therefore, be worthwhile to check with your local and state water agencies regarding the content and safety of the water you use.

Types of Oil

Most cooked meals, and even salads for that matter, use oil in some form or another. Although up to 30 percent (60–65 g) of our dietary needs may be taken as fats (except in very cold environments where more may be needed for thermoregulation of the body), the choice of oil used is important to avoid unhealthy effects. This is a function of the amount of saturated fatty acids in the oil.

The higher the amount of saturated fatty acids in oil, the more likely it is to have a solid consistency, and the higher possibility there is that it will deposit in the blood vessels and increase the risk for high blood pressure and heart diseases. However, the unsaturated fat in the oil may be monounsaturated (MUFA) or polyunsaturated (PUFA). While MUFA lowers the bad cholesterol selectively, PUFA lowers both the good and the bad cholesterol without discrimination. Of the 30 percent of calories obtained from fat, 8 percent saturated, 12 percent MUFA and 10 percent PUFA would be a good ratio. Care should be taken to avoid heat exposure while storing oil due to possibility of rancidity. In addition, including food products that contain omega 3 fatty acids such as fish, walnuts, and almonds may enhance heart and brain health. Some examples of the amounts of fatty acids in different oils are given below:

Composition of different Oils

Oil	Saturated	MUFA	PUFA
Canola	6%	62%	32%
Safflower	10%	13%	77%
Sunflower	11%	20%	69%
Corn	13%	25%	62%
Olive	14%	77%	9%
Soybean	15%	24%	61%
Rice bran	20%	47%	33%
Margarine—soft	20%	46%	34%
Butter	65%	30%	4%
Margarine—hard	80%	14%	16%

Chapter 18

How Many Calories?

Calories are the amount of energy contained in a food product. Ideally, we should consume the amount needed by our body so that excesses do not accumulate as fat. A simple and effective way of keeping count of what we need and how much we are getting is to know our caloric demands. We expend energy in the following ways:

1. Basal Energy Expenditure
2. Physical Activity
3. Growth (for children) and Repair
4. Dietary Waste

In an adult male, this roughly adds up to 2,300 to 2,900 kcal/day and in an adult woman, it comes to 1,900 to 2,200 kcal/day. The lower end of the range is for the less physically active, while the upper end of the range is for people whose work involves more manual labor. For example, if you are a young woman who works on the computer most of the day, your caloric needs will probably be around 1,900 kcal/day, while one with a job that requires physical labor can burn more calories.

The American Heart Association gives an estimate of caloric need for an individual as follows:

1. Basal Calories =   Weight in pounds X 10
2. Activity Calories =   Weight in pounds X 3 (For mild activity)
                                 Weight in pounds X 5 (For moderate act)
                                 Weight in pounds X 8 (For heavy activity)
3. Total Calories[27] =   Basal + Activity

(Use 10 percent less than Total Calories if age is greater than fifty years.)

It has been recommended that an individual derive about 55 percent of the caloric requirement from carbohydrates and a maximum of 30 percent of energy from fat (although I personally feel that this amount should be lower; diets as low as 10 percent have shown to be safe). The rest is made up by protein consumption.

Again, these needs will change with changes in body physiology. In the case of pregnancy, during which the metabolic demands of the body are increased and the growth of tissues is needed (as also in growing children), the caloric needs are higher (an extra 200–300 kcal per day). On the other hand, with advancing age, the body metabolism slows down and there is a tendency toward diminished physical activity; therefore, caloric needs are lower.

The importance of this information lies in understanding the basic reason for weight problems. If an individual consumes roughly the same amount of calories that his body needs and expends, his weight will remain stable. When he or she consumes calories in excess of what his body can use, the extra calories get converted into fat and are stored in the body. Similarly, if an individual consumes fewer calories than he or she needs, the body starts using the stored body fat to meet its metabolic needs. Simply put, if you eat too much, you increase stored body fat; if you restrict your food or eat the right kind, you lose body fat. This is probably the most important concept to understand and apply if appropriate body composition is to be gained.

---

[27]Try the following website to calculate individual calories:
URL- http://www.ahealthyme.com/topic/calneed

Chapter 19

Our Weight

Our body contour is essentially a function of the thickness of muscle and fat that is underneath our skin and over our bony frame. A rough idea about how much one should weigh can be deduced from height. This is because muscle mass and tissues—including the needed fat reserve—are of a certain ratio to the height of the skeletal system.

A scientific basis of such an evaluation is given by the calculation of body mass index (BMI).[28] This index is calculated by dividing the weight in kilograms by the square of the height in meters.

BMI= Weight (kg) / Height squared (m²)

A value between 18.5 and 24.9 corresponds to the normal range. A BMI of less than 18.5 is considered underweight. A BMI of more than 25.0 falls in the category of overweight, and more than 30 qualifies as obesity. A BMI value above 40 is considered severe obesity, and this poses significant health hazards. Individuals with BMIs above 40, or more than 200% relative weight, have a tenfold higher risk of death than someone of normal weight.

---

[28]Calculations available on the following website:
URL- http://www.nhlbisupport.com/bmi/

Concerns with Obesity

"Your body is the baggage you must carry through life. The more the excess baggage the shorter the trip."
~A. Glasgow

Why should we try to be within a certain range of weight? Should it be for the aesthetics and physical acceptance? But what if we don't care about how others perceive us? What if we are happy enough within ourselves that we do not need to concern ourselves with the aesthetics of the physical form? That is probably the last reason one should try and achieve ideal weight. Avoiding multiple problems and diseases that come with obesity should be the main motivation for working toward an acceptable body form. Here are just a few; these are best read more than once so that they will stay in our memory for a lifetime!

1. Diabetes: Increased deposition of fat in the internal organs— specifically the liver—tends to increase the resistance to insulin action. Insulin is a hormone that closely regulates sugar in the blood; therefore, obesity interferes with its action and causes raised blood sugar, a condition called NIDDM (Non Insulin Dependent Diabetes Mellitus), or type 2 diabetes. The chronic elevation of blood sugar plays havoc with body physiology. It can cause problems of hypertension (high blood pressure), kidney disease, and retinal dysfunction (severe eye disorders), just to name a few.

2. Hypertension: Excessive fat in the body is stored in different parts of the body depending on the age and sex of an individual. Particularly in men and post-menopausal women, this tends to be in the waist area and the viscera (internal organs). The increased circulation of free fatty acids tends to also cause fat deposition in the blood vessels, which structurally distorts them and makes them more rigid, resulting in abnormalities of blood pressure.

3. Cardiovascular disease: One of the most concerning places that fat may deposit is the arteries (blood vessels) that supply blood to vital organs like the heart and brain. If there is excessive deposition of lipids in these vessels, the blood supply gets compromised either due to narrowing of the vessels or slowing of blood flow, which can cause clot formation. This may become so significant that parts of the affected organ may die from lack of oxygen and nutrition, causing conditions such as heart attack and stroke. Of all deaths in the U.S., heart attacks are the leading cause of death.

4. Arthritis: Our joints are structured to carry a certain weight. With increasing weight, the joints work harder and the bony surfaces are pushed closer together, destroying the cartilage that covers them. This sets up a reaction called inflammation, which further destroys the joint surfaces, resulting in Osteoarthirits. The pain from the disorder prevents a person from mobilizing, and therefore physical activity decreases. With decreasing activity, the amount of calories that are burned lower, and more calories are stored as fat, resulting in more weight gain. And hence a vicious cycle ensues. More weight, more joint problems, less exercise, more weight.

5. Others: Obese individuals tend to have higher incidence of gall bladder disease, breathlessness, sleep apnea, reflux esophagitis (heartburn), gallstones, and gout. Some studies have suggested that there may also be a higher risk of cancer (breast, uterus, and colon), fertility impairment, cystic ovary disease and chronic back pain.

One can see that the body is intended to be a certain way. The consequences of obesity are problematic, painful, and they put an individual at increased risk for premature death. Clearly, no well-being is possible unless we attend to this issue. Once we know what an appropriate body structure is and why it is so important to aim for it, it is time to figure out how to achieve it.

Why Do We Become Obese?

One out of every three (about 30 percent) Americans, about 97 million people, are either overweight or obese. In some populations, specifically African-Americans and Hispanics, this problem is as high as two out of four (50 percent). This is probably the major reason for the alarming increase in the associated co-morbidities, such as diabetes and cardiovascular accidents.

Obesity is considered to be due to a combination of genetic and environmental causes. Identical twins raised in different environments tend to have similar body compositions, and immigrants from underdeveloped countries tend to show higher BMIs after adapting to the American lifestyle. Some of my own research in rats regarding eating behavior led me to discover that there are some peptides in the brain that may be responsible for increasing feeding desire. One such peptide is Neuropeptide Y. This protein element is found in much higher quantities in the feeding centers of the brains (Hypothalamus) in rats that are naturally obese than those that are not. Their progeny (subsequent generations) have the same tendency and peptide concentrations in their hypothalamic regions. On the other hand, a lean variety of rats have lower quantities of this protein in their brains and are easily satisfied with smaller quantities of food. Interestingly, when we injected this peptide into the brains of baby rats that exhibited poor weight gain, their weight increased much more rapidly! More recently, a gene designated ob and its peptide leptin have been thought to be associated with obesity in rodents, probably in association with other genes and their products.

Clearly, obesity is a multi-factorial problem; it probably has an underlying genetic or inherited component with environmental factors adding fuel to the fire. The degree of influence each of these factors plays in the overall picture varies in individuals. A tendency to have an excessive desire to eat, decreased body metabolism, decreased physical activity, and the consumption of food with high fat content probably all contribute in inducing and maintaining this condition. These above mentioned items may also be contributing factors to the increase in weight with aging in addition to decreasing basic metabolic rate.

In simple terms, obesity is the net result of more calories going in than coming out!

"Apple" and "Pear" Obesity

For those among who feel they are obese, take a moment and look at yourselves closely. The excess fat deposits in our bodies tend to be concentrated so as to produce two different types of body shapes. First, it may be distributed mainly in the lower part of our bodies, i.e., mainly upper thighs, hips, and lower abdomen, resulting in a bottom-heavy, or pear–shaped, body. This is more common in women and is less likely to be associated with cardiovascular disease, although the other complications of obesity still exist. Second, the excess fat may be distributed in the middle parts of the body, i.e., in the waist and flank area, or spread all over, causing one to have a rounded appearance, or an apple-shaped body. This is more commonly seen in men, and they tend to have a higher risk for hypertension and heart diseases due to lipid deposits in the blood vessels around the heart. Medically, this is measured as a waist-to-hip ratio, and values more than one for men and more than 0.8 for women are reasons for concern. It is, therefore, imperative that before embarking on strenuous exercise plans, evaluation by a physician through clinical and laboratory indices be undertaken.

Chapter 20

Correcting the Weight Problem

Correcting a weight problem is not unlike adjusting a bank balance. Regardless of the cause of the problem and the fat distribution, the treatment of excessive weight is essentially based on two principles:

1. Lower caloric intake

2. Increase energy expenditure

In practical terms, eat right, eat less, and burn calories. It is also important to keep in mind that an individual's attitude, mood, and stress level contribute greatly to his or her "excess baggage." This is probably a function of eating habits, seeking comfort in food, and the body's hormonal balance.

The majority of weight loss tends to be achieved by diet control, while the other aspect of correcting the weight is discussed in detail in the respective sections on attitude, thoughts, habits, and stress, with the other major component being exercising. It is helpful to consider dietary measures in two stages: an initial intensive approach and a subsequent lifestyle change.

Two Stages of Diet Correction

To allow easy application and achieve timely results, diet correction for an overweight condition can be considered in two stages.

1. Reduction phase

2. Maintenance phase

The reduction phase involves following dietary restrictions with discipline and dedication till the desired weight is reached. Following that, the maintenance phase is comprised of making healthy changes in eating choices.

1. Reduction Phase

In the reduction phase, strict diet control needs to be implemented until target weight or healthy Body Mass Index is reached. This often means that the caloric intake should be 60–70 percent of what may be permissible for a person of ideal weight. For example, if a woman with a desk job is initiating weight loss, her daily caloric consumption should be roughly 2,000 kcal in a day if she does not have a weight problem. In the reduction phase for an individual with a similar lifestyle and a weight problem, the calories consumed in a day should be between 1,200 and 1,400. How do you do that without starving? How does one fill up and enjoy this process so that one never needs to go back to scale-breaking weights?

The main thrust in the initial stages is to find healthy alternatives and strategies to curb appetite. In essence, this means using the simple but effective method of filling up with food items that provide lower calories. As previously discussed, the maximum amount of calories per gram is provided by fat. Also, fat that is consumed is more easily converted to body stores than protein and carbohydrates. Therefore, ensuring low-fat content in food (less than three grams for snacks) is the initial crucial step.

The second step should be finding low-calorie food items that are filling yet enjoyable. For example, if one is craving hot dogs and decides to eat one, this is how much it can cost in terms of calories:

Meat (140 kcal) + Bread (80 kcal) + Mayonnaise (60 kcal) + Dressing (40 kcal) = 320 kcal.

On the other hand, if we replace all those components with *low-fat ingredients*, we can reduce the number of calories significantly:

Meat (40) + Bread (40) + Mayonnaise (20) + Dressing (20) = 120 Cal.

In analysis, the realization is that we can eat a meal with almost a third of the calories that we would have consumed if we were not careful. Once we start paying attention to this on a regular basis, we will realize that just choosing the right food will make all the difference! So, while we are still determined and motivated, we should look around and check all the food items within our reach, at home, at work, and in the car and replace those with low-fat, low-calorie items.

The final step is discovering the power of water to help reduce your intake by almost 30 percent (In a personal experiment, I noticed that if I had a glass of water before a meal, I needed to eat one-third less to fill up!). We need about six to eight glasses of water to flush out our wastes and replace our fluid losses. But water (room temperature), if taken before meals, also adds to the stomach content, reducing the capacity available for other food products.

If we were to put some of these concepts in easy, effective steps, the initial simple rules would be as follows:

Types of food

- Do not eat desserts (this includes candies and chocolates).

- Do not eat fried food (sorry, no fries!).

- Maintain a low-fat, low-salt, high-protein, and high-fiber diet (fat free cheese, soy products, salads [with 0–20 calorie dressings], skim milk, fruits that are not extremely sweet, low sugar cereal, water bagels, lentils, low-fat meat, and bread).

- Keep low-fat snacks within reach in case you get extremely hungry.

(All items should have less than three grams of fat.)

Filling up

- Drink six to eight glasses of water or other zero-calorie fluids each day (one glass of room-temperature water before meals).

- Sit down and enjoy food without any distractions.
  (Avoid reflex eating, or eating while engaged in another activity, such as reading, watching TV, or watching a movie. Eating should be done in response to hunger and addressed that way.)

- Chew food well.
  (Spend time with food and make it quality time! Do justice to your food so that it is broken down into small particles, preferably a paste, that the body can benefit from. In essence, chewing each bite well is as important as choosing the right food. You should feel tired of eating by the time you are done so that you think twice before you pop something in your mouth to "just get a taste.")

- Eat when you are hungry, or in intervals of every four hours.
(The stomach is empty approximately four hours after eating.)

- Take only as much food as makes you comfortable without making you feel full. Some people benefit from wearing tight-fitting clothing around the waist to get that snug and can't-have-any-more feeling!

- Replace activities involving eating out with healthy alternatives, such as walks, gym, bowling, swimming, etc.

- Beware of the places where you eat.
(Most restaurant food is tasty because it is greasy. If you have no other choice, find healthy alternatives or ask for diet entrées. I found a simple solution in some fast food restaurants at which my kids like to eat by asking them to make a grilled/baked chicken or fish sandwich without mayonnaise or any sauces. Other options may be to eat the meat without the bread.)

- Additional help will come from increasing physical exertion, which will help burn more calories, mobilize stored fat, and increase your metabolic rate. The methods of exercise are so many that it deserves complete attention, and therefore a separate section is devoted to it. In addition to other forms of exercises, the single most important exercise to include in the reduction phase is: Shake your head from side to side when offered the wrong food or food at the wrong time!

- Maintain a positive attitude, address stress, and avoid using food as a comfort substitute.

Weight loss should be slow and steady. Overly rapid weight loss is undesirable because it can cause loss of lipid support in some internal organs, such as the kidneys, and it may cause floating kidney syndrome. It is also associated with sagging skin and rebound weight increase. Initial weight loss is usually very encouraging, but it slows down after the first few weeks. This is primarily a result of some water loss as fat stores are mobilized. Consistent weight loss until you reach your desired BMI should be the goal.

Examples of Meals during the Reduction Phase

Time of Day	Meal	Cal
MORNING	Warm water with lemon with or without few drops of honey	0-10
BREAKFAST	Glass of warm skim milk	80
	Fat free Cheese or Banana or ½ Bagel or Boiled Egg without yellow	100
SNACK (Optional)	Water	0
	Low fat free snack of less than 100 Cal (Fruit or Flavored Soy nuts)	100
LUNCH	Water	0
	Salad (watch the fat content in the dressing, low fat toppings)	40
	Bread (low fat)	40
	Chicken Breast grilled	200
SNACK (Optional)	Water	0
	Fat free snack of less than 100 Cal	100
DINNER	Water	0
	Mixed vegetables	100
	Fat free yogurt	100
	Meal (such as Weight watchers frozen cuisines) with about 200 Cal and 3 grams fat	200
	TOTAL	1070

2. Maintenance Phase

Once we have reached the desirable weight, we can switch to a maintenance phase. This essentially means consuming the recommended number of calories for your lifestyle, age, and gender. It is probably better to stay under 90 percent of the caloric requirements for those who have treated their obesity, as there is evidence to suggest that their lipid metabolism and energy expenditure may be lower than normal.

This is the stage during which you can allow yourself a small helping of dessert if you take less of the main menu. As a rule of thumb, I would recommend a portion no bigger than the length of your thumb in width and height for your serving size, and restricted to no more than twice a week.

Appetite issues

There are certain anticipated and unanticipated times during which our appetite tends to be beyond our control. Thanks to the motion of the gut, acid secretions in the stomach, neurochemicals bathing our brain, and changes in the metabolic and endocrinal milieu of our bodies, our perception of hunger is inevitable. Therefore, despite our best of efforts, wisdom, and motivation, we experience pangs of hunger that need to be attended to. Here are some useful strategies that will take care of this problem most of the time:

- If you have to go to a dinner gathering, you will find yourself eating excessively just because you are watching others eat. The entrées served at parties are often high in fat content because the fat makes them taste better. Have a glass of warm milk before you leave, arrive after snacks have already been served, and start your meal with a glass of water.

- Anticipate hunger problems in the premenstrual period. Attend to it by using a zero-calorie filling solution, e.g., drink hot, decaffeinated coffee or tea (try green tea or tea with one small cardamom or a pinch of its powder). Alternatively, drink low-fat soup or lemon tea to fill up. Low-fat yogurt also helps to soothe the stomach and ease mental distress. Sucking on a calcium tablet (like Tums') once or twice a day helps neutralize stomach acid, thereby alleviating hunger pangs. As an added benefit, it helps prevent osteoporosis.

- Many complain that the worst period of hunger pangs tend to be while driving back home after a day's work. Take a water drink or a warm beverage and a banana (a good source of potassium, which helps prevent blood pressure problems) with you and you will feel pretty satisfied by the time you get home.

Chapter 21

Anticipated Problems in Weight Control

Despite the simplicity of the basic concept of regulating calories, why are people not able to correct the highly prevalent problem of excess weight and obesity? Being overweight is a condition that, by current estimates, is affecting close to half the U.S. population. It essentially comes down to having enough determination to overcome the genetic and environmental influences in our lives, the temptation of tasty food, and the influences of sedentary living. Not uncommonly, after becoming knowledgeable about the consequences, people do take the most important step: initiation. They also often achieve some degree of success, but unfortunately, they are often unable to continue with the next important step: staying motivated and determined.

So, how can we ensure that? One essentially needs checkpoints. Whether these are going to be mental or physical depends upon an individual's nature and need for external sources for motivation. Some suggestions are as follows:

Staying Motivated

- Place motivating slogans, such as "You can do it," around yourself (on the bathroom mirror, refrigerator, study desk, car).

- Paste a picture of a very fat person and a well-built person side by side in a drawer that you see every day and write underneath "What is going to be your future?"

- Remind yourself that perfection needs time and patience. Rome was not built in a day; one of the world's wonders, the Taj Mahal, took twenty-two years to be completed

Checkpoints

- Check your weight on Monday, Wednesday, and Friday. If there is persistent gain for three days, start a diet diary.

- Start the program with a friend and share progress on a weekly basis.

- If you have had more than two failures, enroll in a Weight Watchers plan that has a follow-up of at least eighteen months.

Other Treatments for Severe Obesity

In severe obesity (a BMI of more than forty or a relative weight of more than 200 percent), when diet and exercising have failed, there are some other forms of medical and surgical help available. Medications that suppress appetite have been tried, although concerns regarding their addictive nature and the possibility of cardiovascular disease have made them less attractive. More recently, medications that lower fat absorption or increase metabolic rate have begun to be evaluated. Surgical gastric bypass or vertical banding or gastroplasty are occasionally used in extreme cases of obesity, but even then the mainstay of the management is dietary control and physical activity.

Cosmetic removal of fat from some body areas, referred to as liposuction, only offers temporary effects and is easily reversed if the basic essentials of weight control are not followed. A recent discovery regarding the obesity gene has aroused interest in potential gene therapy, but it is likely to take years before we see any benefits from this if we see any at all. Regardless of the method used, these medical procedures are helpful only if they serve as an adjunct to the basic rules of weight control: consume less; burn more calories.

Bottom line: Stick with the basic rules and enjoy good health! Slow and steady wins the race, and don't forget to enjoy the ride!

Chapter 22

Aging and Weight Control

When looking at the pictures of an individual in his or her youth, most people are amazed as to how thin he or she was. Whether it is a change in our hormonal make-up, an alteration in our metabolism, a difference in our feeding practices, or an adaptation to a different lifestyle, this phenomenon appears to affect us sooner or later.

It was probably intended that way by nature to enhance aging and the eventual demise of a being in order to replace them with younger, more effective bodies. But with the superior intelligence of man, this need not be so. In fact, because of the way man has evolved, the skills, knowledge, and experience acquired over the years makes an elder individual more valuable and efficient. Applying the simple measures of appetite control, ingesting the right kinds of food items, and keeping oneself active can help us overcome these natural physical changes.

On the other hand, body-conscious preteens and teenagers need to be cautious about restricting calories, especially proteins, so as not to restrict their growth. More emphasis on physical activities and eating the right types of food is the desired route at this age.

Some simple measures may help us in controlling weight after the age of fifty, when it appears especially difficult to keep within the desirable range. These include the following-

Stay Hydrated

Start your day with a glass of water. Ensure that you take six to eight glasses of salt-free fluids every day without fail. Drink a glass of water before each meal to help avoid overeating.

Be Active after Meals

It is a valid concern for many that after the age of fifty, weight gain is faster despite the same amount of food consumption as before. This may be caused by a decrease in body metabolism. One way to counteract this concern is to increase the body metabolism by staying active. Therefore, eating and sleeping may not be the best practices!

Split the Workout

Another way of optimizing an increase in metabolism may be to exercise twice for thirty minutes versus exercising once for one hour. This would serve to spread the fat utilization period over a longer time; because the body's metabolism would be increased more than once a day, the burning of calories would accordingly be boosted more than once per day.

Type of Food

There are some healthy choices that one can opt for in order to minimize caloric consumption, Choosing fat-free milk instead of low-fat milk, choosing soy products instead of cheese, choosing lean meat instead of regular, etc., may go a long way in lowering the caloric load and resultant unhealthy weight trend.

Healthy Options

Food often serves as a comfort and a default activity for many. Additionally, stress provokes an unconscious feeding reflex that people engage in to find comfort and escape. As one strives to achieve a stress-free state (refer to the section on the mind), this may be less of a concern. Additionally, finding active hobbies can serve as a healthy alternative to eating.

Chapter 23

Supplements

Many compounds called vitamins have been shown to be associated with various important functions in the body. Vitamins are chemicals that are needed in small quantities (milligram or microgram amounts) to serve as adjuncts to certain metabolic functions in the body. These are conventionally divided into categories of fat soluble (vitamins A, D, E, and K) and water soluble (vitamin B complex and vitamin C). More recently, Vitamin H (biotin) and Vitamin P (bioflavonoids) are names given to compounds previously considered part of the vitamin B complex.

The distinction of fat-soluble and water-soluble vitamins is helpful in allowing us to understand that excess amounts of fat-soluble vitamins can be harmful because they can be stored in the body. On the other hand, if excess amounts of water-soluble vitamins are consumed, they tend to be excreted from the body (although very high chronic doses of vitamin C can precipitate as calcium citrate stones in predisposed individuals). Each of these vitamins is distributed in natural food, has a specific function in the body, and is needed in certain amounts. The measure of the amount needed by the body is referred to as DRI (dietary reference intake) or RDA (recommended dietary allowance) by the National Academy of Sciences.

To add to the confusion, there are an even higher numbers of minerals that our body needs. These are usually considered as major (needed in bigger quantities) and minor (small quantities needed) elements. To make things even more complicated, each of these has a specific function, distribution, and recommended allowance! A quick glance at the accompanying chart will help you realize the complexity of these substances!

Vitamins

Vitamin	Function	Food items

Fat-soluble

Vitamin	Function	Food items
Vitamin A	Wound healing Eyes hair and skin repair	Liver, pigmented vegetables, fruits
Vitamin D	Increases absorption of calcium & phosphate, healthy bones and teeth	Fish, liver, dairy, eggs
Vitamin E	Antioxidant, helps trap free radicals in the body	Vegetable oils, nuts, wheat germ, leafy vegetables
Vitamin K	Promotes proteins to help blood clotting and prevent anemia	Leafy green vegetables

$\mathcal{W}$ater-soluble

Vitamin B Complex: Thiamine (B_1)	Co-enzyme for carbohydrate metabolism	Unrefined grains, liver, nuts
Riboflavin (B_2)	Cell metabolism, enzyme actions	Meat, fish, dairy
Niacin	Enzymes for carbohydrate and fat metabolism	Bean, grain, meat
Pyridoxine (B_6)	Co-enzyme Blood production	Poultry, fish eggs, nuts soybeans
Folate	DNA synthesis Blood production	Vegetables, Fruits, liver
Cobalamine (B_{12})	Cofactor in blood production nerve conduction	Meat, dairy, fish
Biotin	Metabolism of fat and carbohydrate	Liver, soy, egg yolk
Pantothenic acid	Component of Co-enzyme A for and carbohydrate hormone synthesis	Whole grain legumes, meats
Vitamin C	Anti-oxidant Wound healing	Fruits Vegetables

Recommended daily allowances and dietary reference intakes are available from the United States Department of Agriculture at the USDA website.[29]

---

[29] URL- http://www.iom.edu/Object.File/Master/7/296/webtablevitamins.pdf

Minerals

Mineral	Function	Food items
Major		
Calcium	Forms bone, teeth needed for nerve and muscle function	Dairy, fish tofu, greens soybeans, broccoli
Phosphorus	Forms bone, teeth needed for metabolic activities	Dairy, meat eggs, nuts, lentils
Magnesium	Needed for cell activities, nerve and muscle actions	Whole grains, nuts, lentils, green leafy vegetables
Minor		
Iron	Blood production	Meat, eggs, poultry, fish, dried fruits, soybeans, cauliflower, green leafy vegetables
Zinc	Enzyme actions, cell growth and repair	Seafood, meat, eggs soybeans, wheat germ, sunflower seeds
Iodine	Thyroid hormone	Seafood, iodized salt

Selenium	Protects cells from oxidants	Seafood, liver, whole grains
Copper	Component of Enzymes and Protein products	Meats, liver seafood, nuts, seeds
Manganese	Metalloenzyme component	Whole grains, tea, cereal,fruits, vegetables
Fluoride	Teeth and bone formation	Water, tea, marine fish
Chromium	Glucose balance	Brewer's Yeast, Calf liver, Cheese
Molybdenum	Enzyme constituent	Milk, beans bread,cereal

Recommended daily allowances and dietary reference intakes are available from the United States Department of Agriculture at the USDA website.[30]

---

[30] URL- http://www.iom.edu/Object.File/Master/7/294/0.pdf

It is apparent that the list is exhaustive and overwhelming. Take a deep breath and do not panic. Remember, we are here to make life simple and yet healthy. We could spend the rest of our lives trying to make sure we take these in the right amounts and have not time left to do anything else! Here is the easy way that works.

- Try to attend to the basic rules of eating, which were mentioned before. Eating a variety of food from each food category helps provide most of the vitamins and elements

- Eat fresh fruits and lightly cooked vegetables since they contain water-soluble vitamins that can be destroyed by excessive heat.

- Consider a multivitamin and multimineral supplement in case you are unable to ensure your intake of a healthy variety of food products every day. This can be in the form of over-the-counter tablets or capsules, such as Centrum˙ A-Z (or other reputed and tested products), and taken two to three times a week. I usually take these on Monday, Wednesday, and Friday and keep the bottle on the breakfast table to remind the family to take them. This way we are able to replenish any deficiencies and avoid toxicity from overdose (by not taking them every day in addition to what we are getting from diet). Many of my friends and relatives now live by this ritual with good effect!

Additional Supplements

There has been some recent discussion in medical literature regarding the use of certain vitamins and minerals to prevent medical conditions. One such recommendation that has served us well has been the use of vitamin C for alleviating viral respiratory infections. I use 1,000 milligrams of vitamin C (two 500 mg tablets) for three days at the start of any viral or respiratory infection, and have usually avoided suffering. Increased intake of other anti-oxidants, as found in grapes, berries, and vegetable-and-chicken soup, may also help us deal with illnesses better. At the time of seasonal change, when most of the viral infections tend to occur, we take these for prevention once or twice a week. This may have an added advantage of preventing cardiac conditions, and may even prevent cancers, as has been suggested by some researchers, although this is still debated.[31]

For women of menstruating age, it may serve well to take iron supplements for the first three days of the cycle. Growing children, pregnant women and the elderly should pay special heed to their calcium intake to avoid problems with bone density. I have also found the consumption of calcium (1,000 mg or two 500 mg tablets) to be conducive to sleep when feeling overwhelmed or stressed. In fact, taking these in the premenstrual period may help alleviate symptoms of irritability (try green tea in the morning and evening and calcium at night for the three most distressing days in the cycle). Although the exact reason for this is unclear, it may be because calcium exists in the body in an ionic form and helps stabilize the cell membrane ionic potential that exists in all cells and is especially useful in nerves and muscles for impulse conduction and contraction, thereby calming the nerves. It is not surprising then that calcium deficiency leads to a condition marked by excessive twitching and spasms. Families with history of hypertension need to keep their salt intake low, as it may contribute to high blood pressure, especially in African and Asian populations.

Different elements of the vitamin B complex, especially thiamine (B_1), niacin (B_6), and pyridoxine (B_{12}), may have neuroprotective effects. It is currently debatable as to whether they improve brain functioning, but their deficiency is definitely associated with neurological symptoms. VISP (Vitamin Intervention in Stroke Prevention) is a research effort evaluating the use of certain B vitamins in preventing stroke. More recently, scientific information has found that the adequate intake of folic acid in a woman of child-bearing age reduces her chances of having a baby with neural tube defect. Given this background, I take B complex and folic acid supplements once a week.

The antioxidant properties of vitamin E were a hot discovery in the 1980s. This raised hope for use of this vitamin in the prevention

---

[31] URL- http://www.nutritionj.com/content/2/1/7

of malignant diseases and possibly as an anti-aging aid. Although this vitamin is needed in only small quantities, taking a vitamin E supplement once a week may eventually be beneficial.

Intakes low in sodium (less than 2.5 grams of sodium or 6.0 grams of sodium chloride (salt)—minimum of 0.5 g of salt) and high in potassium (this is found in fresh fruits and unprocessed vegetables; it has a daily requirement of 50 mEq or 2.0 grams) may serve as prevention against hypertension in some ethnic groups, primarily Asians and Native Americans. In a nutshell, you should consume plenty of fruits and vegetables and adhere to a low-salt diet.

Simply put, it may be worthwhile to take a supplement every day at a time one is most likely to remember, if our diets are sometimes lacking. I prefer to do this after breakfast, and my own week looks something like this:

Day of the Week	Supplements *
Mon	Multi-vitamin and multi-mineral (A-Z)
Tue	B Complex, Calcium
Wed	Multi-vitamin and multi-mineral (A-Z)
Th	Folic Acid, Calcium
Fri	Multi-vitamin and multi-mineral (A-Z)
Sat	Vitamin C, Calcium
Sun	Vitamin E

(*This schedule is per the opinion and practice of the author. These supplements are available at any pharmacy store. Chose a reputed and tested product)

Some recent studies have brought to light the possible usefulness of drinking red wine in lowering the incidence of heart diseases (atherosclerosis and myocardial infarction). This may be due to the presence antioxidants, such as phenols (resveratrol in red wine), present in these alcoholic beverages, and is believed to explain the "French Paradox" of low heart attacks despite diet rich in fat. However, the excessive consumption of alcohol defeats any such advantage (death and disability due to accidents, diseases such as liver cirrhosis, nutritional deficiencies). Therefore if alcohol is consumed it is best to restrict it to less than three to four drinks a week (to avoid an addictive pattern), with each drink being no more than six ounces. Women planning pregnancy should avoid any form of alcohol to prevent harmful effects on the fetus. More importantly, similar benefit may be obtained by eating a healthy diet, regular intake of antioxidant vegetables and fruits especially grapes, and following a dedicated schedule of exercising. Therefore "health benefit" should not necessarily be construed as an excuse to drink!

Protein Supplements

There has been some recent discussion in the health industry about the benefits of protein supplements in the form of protein hydrolysates, amino acids, l-glutamine, and carnitine. Since an adult male requires close to sixty grams of protein per day, and more so for the exercising person, these needs may not met unless one makes a special effort to take in adequate protein. Additionally, there have been some claims that protein supplementation enhances the production of growth hormone in the body, which is associated with delaying aging by enhancing tissue repair. The data, however, is inconclusive, and concern regarding product constituents and effects of excess consumption should be considered. Fascinating combination supplements are being scientifically engineered under the guidance of physicians by some companies such as ViSalus Sciences®.

Enzyme Supplements

Some individuals are unable to effectively digest certain food products containing lactose (milk-containing products). This results in flatulence, and occasionally, diarrhea. Use of a lactase enzyme supplement can help alleviate these symptoms.

Other food products that contain branching or complex sugars, such as legumes and broccoli, can cause discomfort and embarrassing gas passage. Supplemental enzymes that have the enzyme alpha galactosidase, such as Beano˙, may be beneficial. Other uses of supplemental enzymes are being explored, but these supplements should be taken only after consultation with a doctor since some interact with other medications.

Enzymes to aid digestion are also found in certain plants. Two commonly used, natural, enzyme-containing fruits are pineapple (enzyme Bromelain), and papaya (enzyme Papain). These fruits contain enzymes that hydrolyze certain proteins and may be useful to consume with high-protein products such as meat, eggs, or legumes. Dr. Edward Howell's (physician and researcher) book *Enzyme Nutrition* has extensive information on his research and theories of how enzymes can affect health and longevity.

Chapter 24

Life without Addictions

---

*"Is life so wretched? Isn't it rather your hands, which are
too small, your vision which is muddled? You are the one
who must grow up."*
~Dag Hammarskjold

There is a natural tendency in every human being to seek pleasure
and avoid pain. Whether these are physical pains or mental agonies,
real or imagined, our survival instincts compel us to comfort
ourselves in one way or another. The mentally stronger among us
are able to find this healing within themselves; others may have
the advantage of an effective family or social support. Some others
may seek help from appropriate agencies, be they medical or social,
to enable them to return to a normal physical and mental state of
functioning. Unfortunately, a concerning number of people (which
seems to be increasing daily) fall into the trap of using mind-altering
drugs to shake them out of their despair. Sadly enough, this is also
sometimes the result of curiosity and experimenting (especially
among teenagers) with these highly addictive drugs.

What are Drugs?

Addictive drugs, also known medically as abusive substances, are
psychoactive (act on the brain) compounds that alter the mental frame
of an individual. They alter the perception, mood, feelings, and even
behavior, sometimes to the degree where an individual has no idea as

to how he or she is acting. These compounds are classified as either stimulants (e.g. nicotine, marijuana) or depressants (e.g. alcohol) or hallucinogens (e.g. LSD). Regardless of the category, they tend to make a person perceive his situation and environment in a distorted way, essentially throwing a curtain over that person's mind to hide the troubling truth. In addition to the alterations in the thought process, these substances affect one's feelings and emotions. They also cause a person to suffer poor coordination and increased reaction time. In addition, there are changes in the physiological parameters of the body, such as increased heart rate and alterations in blood pressure, which can, in some cases, cause severe medical problems, such as stroke (and possibly paralysis) and the predisposition to angina and myocardial infarction (heart attacks).

What's the Problem?

The most unfortunate part of these drugs is that despite placing an individual in an apparent euphoric mood, they make an individual nonfunctional, which disables an individual from undertaking appropriate action toward remedying the underlying problem. If anything at all, it takes away any potential chances of recovery because overall, the person's performance and behavior deteriorates. To add fuel to the fire, as the effects of the drug wear off, there are neurochemical changes in parts of the brain that force a person to seek more of the addictive psychoactive substance.

In addition, physiological changes in the body, such as sweating, headaches, and vomiting, that are caused by the withdrawal from some of these drugs result in profound and intolerable symptoms, which again compels an individual to take more of the drug. This sets up a wicked vicious cycle of addiction, poor performance, worsening of the underlying problem, and the need for more drugs.

Additionally, each drug has its own significant health hazard to deal with. Smoking, for example, carries a high risk of lung cancers, hypertension, and coronary heart disease. Alcohol attacks the liver, predisposing an individual to chronic liver disease (cirrhosis) and liver cancer. Cocaine is capable of inducing the constriction of blood vessels, causing sudden strokes. Also, the lack of attention to the dietary requirements displayed by the addicted individuals sets them up for nutritional deficiencies, causing anemia and neuropathies.

Poor physical and mental health compromises an individual's performance and capability of retaining his or her job. Add to this the falling socioeconomic status of the individual and the need for more money to buy the drug, and it is easy to see why crime and prostitution are usual eventual accompaniments. A recent analysis brought to our attention the fact that if the prison population continues to rise at this staggering rate, the U.S. will see more people locked up in jails than outside by 2053!

Why the addiction ?

By applying the advances in science, it has been possible to understand why and how these drugs would get a person hooked, which sometimes happens with the first dose. Essentially, most recreational drugs stimulate the reward system of the brain by either releasing or preventing the uptake of a neurochemical called dopamine in the limbic system. This stimulated circuit, located in the hippocampus of the central nervous system, is responsible for a feeling of well-being in an individual.

Activities like eating good food, exercising, being with friends, and watching an enjoyable movie are all capable of providing a person with a similar feeling of well-being. Unfortunately, with the use of drugs, two untoward side effects occur. Firstly, they destroy some dopamine receptors with each use so that more and more stimulus or drug is needed to provide the same feeling of pleasure. Secondly, a memory is created in the mood- and behavior-controlling parts of the brain that compels an individual to consume these destructive agents.

With the help of MRI (magnetic resonance imaging) and PET (positive emission tomography) scanning, it has been shown that these effects may indeed last a long time, so an individual who was addicted to these substances in the past can easily fall prey to relapse in moments of stress.

What can we do?

Clearly, if you are an individual of any intelligence, care for your future, and have never tried drugs, you are a lucky person. Knowing that these substances are a sure way to hell on earth, you should pledge never to even be near them. You may cross paths with colleagues and so-called friends who will try to tempt you to at least try a drug once. These are people who are already living in a rapidly deteriorating lifestyle and are hoping to pull some more people down into the hellhole. But remember: even a single dose can take you far from yourself with nothing but devastation ahead. Sometimes a simple "no" does not sound strong enough to these people who, for social or financial reasons, push others into such addictions. Your best bet is to avoid these people totally, and if possible, to send help their way.

On the other hand, if you happen to be among the ones who are already in the grip of this devastating problem, you need to seek help now. Do not allow another day to go by while these highly caustic elements are destroying your body, mind, and spirit and robbing you and your family of a happy, healthy, and peaceful existence. This help should consist of a strong and caring medical system, a loving and supportive social group, and most importantly, a determined will on your own part to put an end to this life of decay. (I highly recommend reading the section on mental health with special emphasis on attitude and stress relief.) There are many agencies you can contact about this problem, including your own physician or nearby hospital. A call to 1-800-NCA-CALL can get you all the help you need if you do not know which direction to head. (This number is for the National Council of Alcohol and Drug Dependence; their website is www.ncadd.org) Or simply walk into the emergency room of a nearby hospital and ask for help. As Christian Barnard has so correctly put it,

"Suffering isn't ennobling, recovery is."

Society has woven within itself many vices under the excuse of convenience and socialization. We have become very comfortable with the use of some addictive and mind-altering chemicals in our daily lives without necessarily labeling them as drugs. Nicotine (cigarette-smoking), alcohol, and caffeine are among them. These seemingly benign elements can have significant and serious implications. Hypertension, nutritional deficiencies, alterations in brain and body chemistry, and declines in physical and mental capabilities without their use should make us realize their harmful effects and motivate us to eliminate their interference in achieving well-being. Consider the information from the American Medical Association stating that the leading causes of death in 2000 were tobacco (435,000 deaths—18.1% of total U.S. deaths), and alcohol consumption (85,000 deaths—3.5% of total U.S. deaths).[32] This is in addition to many other deaths from heart disease, liver failure, and stroke that are due to the side effects of these toxic substances.

The rules to obtain freedom from these dependences are simple:

1. Obtaining knowledge and understanding of the harmful effects of drugs
   (Some of the above information should help.)

---

[32] URL- http://www.stopaddiction.com/narconon_alcohol_deaths.html#

2. Developing the determination and motivation to end addiction
   (See the section on thought and action in this book.)

3. Planning a strategy and its execution
   (It may be cold turkey if the addiction is early and mild, or it may be staged with step by step decreases over a defined time period to end the addiction if it is long-term and mild to moderate. In case of moderate to severe addictions, medical help with possible pharmacotherapy is warranted.)

4. Creating checkpoints
   (Use self-indicators and help from close confidants to monitor progress and intervene with appropriate measures in case of failures.)

5. Use of support system
   (Both internal, as in the mental and spiritual sections of this book with special emphasis on stress relief and building self-awakening, as well as external, as in friends and family helping find new meaning in life, support systems are available. Not-for-profit organizations like NCADD can help refer people to appropriate de-addiction agencies.)

Chapter 25

Toxins in Our Environment

Unfortunately, just looking at the calories and protein in the food we ingest is not good enough nowadays. There are contaminants, both biological and chemical, that are capable of affecting our health adversely. Being aware of these toxins can help us prevent their short- and long-term negative consequences on our health. One may ask why some of these toxins are FDA (Food and Drug Administration) approved. Essentially, although animal data exists, there is paucity of conclusive studies in humans. Also, many of these agents are used in small quantities, and some are used in diet drinks, so it is felt that the chances of dying from obesity are much higher than the negative effects of these substances. However, it is important that we be aware of these controversies and avoid these products whenever possible. This is not a complete list, as new information always alters and adds to our current understanding.

Chemical Toxins

A common ingredient in the diet drinks, sweeteners, and sugar-free gums is a chemical called aspartame, which is methyl ester of a combination of two amino acids: aspartic acid and phenylalanine. On metabolism in the body it breaks down to form methanol and eventually formaldehyde, which are potential nerve toxins. This product has been shown in animals to affect the neurons in the brain, with concerns of seizures, brain damage and tumors. Although there is no firm direct evidence in humans as yet, it is better to

135

avoid sweeteners in situations where a medical condition prohibits consuming sugar.

Saccharine, another product used as an artificial sweetener, has been linked with bladder cancer in animals. Its carcinogenic potential in humans has not been established, but it may be best avoided or restricted in quantity.

MSG[33], or monosodium glutamate, used often in Chinese food for flavoring, has been associated with neurological symptoms. Many restaurants now offer MSG-free entrees.

Preservatives, such as nitrates and nitrites in the meats, have also been incriminated in malignancies in animals, compelling many consumers to seek organic foods.

Mercury and pesticide wastes in seafood have become an increasing concern due to industrial dumping. Choosing ocean fish and not very fatty fishes may circumvent this problem somewhat.

Another environmental pollutant that can have significant negative consequences on our health is lead. Surprisingly, in addition to chipping wall paint in old homes, lead may get into your food if you use ceramics and lead from some third-world countries. More recently, high levels of this element have been found in some imported candles. So check the labels before you sit down for your aromatherapy!

Check the Container

Recently, concern has been raised about cellular toxins such as diethylhexyadipate (DHEA) and dioxin released from polyvinyl chloride (PVC) when heating plastic containers. This may especially

---

[33] URL- http://www.foodandhealth.com/cpecourses/msg.php

be the case with food containing fat, as dioxin easily migrates and dissolves in it. Additionally, the use of plastic wraps not designated for the microwave and containing PVC may cause similar concern while heating food. Also, chemicals called phthalates are sometimes used to make plastics less brittle and can potentially interfere with hormonal actions. Although controversy surrounds this issue, it may, be best to avoid heating food in plastic containers, or foam containers for that matter, to enjoy a toxin-free meal.

Biological

Eating fresh food and washing thoroughly before eating are simple rules that can help you to avoid microbial, pesticide, or preservative overdose. Meat, such as cold cuts, has been known to accumulate high levels of bacteria even while under refrigeration within a few days of opening the packages. Sometimes these are capable of causing significant illness in the consumer. Freezing items that are not going to be consumed in a short time may be a healthier choice. In case previously refrigerated food needs to be eaten, it may be a good idea to heat the food well before consuming it.

Have it Germ Free

It was during the school year that my youngest child was in second grade when I realized the increased frequency with which he was getting colds and throat infections. Knowing that bacteria and viruses get into the body more commonly through dirty hands and decaying food than by any other method, I arranged for him to get fresh food each day, and I gave him a bottle of sanitizer because he told me he wasn't getting enough time to wash his hands. That was the last time I saw him getting sick that year. Now we carry a bottle of sanitizer with us all the time (in the car, bag, etc.) and avoid eating cold food in restaurants where adequate health precautions are not taken (gloves, hair nets, etc.).

Brushing our teeth before we put anything in our mouth after waking up may sound trivial to many, but unfortunately this is overlooked by some. When your mouth smells foul, your breath is teeming with germs. Ideally, we should brush after each meal, but rinsing with water after each meal and brushing after waking up and before sleeping will go a long way to ensure the company of healthy teeth that will help digest our well-chosen food. In addition, flossing at least before bedtime further ensures removing food stuck in our teeth that is bound to decay and cause bacterial growth and tooth erosion.

Electrical

There has been increasing concern regarding the effect of prolonged exposure to excessive electromagnetic fields due to some houses being built in close proximity to high-intensity electrical power lines and also from use of some appliances. This continues to be a controversial topic, with some studies suggesting a risk versus others showing none. The National Institute for Occupational Health and Safety (NIOSH) periodically reviews the data and releases their workgroup members' opinions at their website.[34]

While this issue continues to be debated, I consider it worthwhile to avoid residing in homes just next to power lines and to avoid the prolonged use of electrical appliances close to the body (cell phones, laptops).

---

[34] URL- http://www.cdc.gov/niosh/topics/emf/

Chapter 26

Check it Out

Despite our attention to many issues relating to the physical body, not every aspect can be analyzed on the basis of body weight and consumption. Heredity and unknown environmental influences are capable of altering the body balances and causing diseases.

In particular, hypertension, diabetes, the risk of heart attacks, stroke, and cancer need to be screened periodically. Early diagnosis of or early recognition of any predisposition to these conditions helps improve the outcome and lower the risk of complications and death. So when was the last time you saw your physician, or do you even have one? If cost is a concern, check out the community physicians' clinics and get yourself checked out. In addition to a general checkup and evaluation of blood pressure, requesting serum cholesterol, LDL, HDL, and blood sugar (and hemoglobin for the menstruating women) testing will help in fine-tuning.

Blood Pressure	Less than 120/80
Serum Cholesterol	Less than 200 mg/dl
Low-Density Lipoproteins	Less than 100 mg/dl
High-Density Lipoproteins	40 mg/dl or higher
Total Cholesterol: HDL	Less than 5:1
Blood Sugar	Fasting 70–100 mg/dl After meal < 140 mg/dl

Hemoglobin	Man	13–17 g/dl
	Woman	12–15 g/dl

Other tests include blood electrolyte testing and liver, kidney, and thyroid function tests.

(Homocysteine, Lipoprotein (a) levels and Treadmill Stress test with EKG monitoring can also be evaluated to determine risk for cardiovascular disease particularly in individuals with strong family history of heart attacks.)

Energizing Activity

Chapter 27

Activity for Fitness

"How do you live a long life? Take a two-mile walk every morning before breakfast."
~Harry S. Truman, U.S. president
(on his eightieth birthday)

The one aspect of a healthy existence that cannot be emphasized enough is indulging in appropriate activity. There is an increasing amount of scientific data supporting the benefits of exercise, making this one of the most essential aspects of healthy living. A large, prospective study from Dallas involving more than 9,000 men showed that indulging in moderate exercise for five years decreases death from all causes and decreases heart diseases. Other studies have shown improvements in vital organ systems, including the heart, lungs, muscles, and bones. Weight maintenance, the prevention of depression, and even the prevention of cancer have all been associated with the benefits of exercising.[35]

Life, for most of us, is extremely busy and often physically tiring enough that the last thing we want to add is extra muscle work. The idea of coming home and flopping on the couch and allowing a TV show to put us into a deep slumber often sounds like the best idea for the evening. For many of us, that may not be feasible, as we return to our homes to run more errands for the family, for the house, and for the kids; the list just does not seem to end.

---

[35] URL- http://circ.ahajournals.org/cgi/content/full/94/4/857

Ironically, my return of enthusiasm toward structured physical exercise started as an attempt to gain more energy. I was often tired by the time I made it home, and then attending to the needs of my family and household left me totally exhausted, and as a result, frustrated. It was at this time that a friend of mine, who was always on the go, asked me if I was interested in joining her for early morning walks. My liking for this individual prompted me to start this "not-so-sure" endeavor.

I was astonished by the results of this self-inflicted experiment. Before the end of the week, I was lighter on my feet, could keep up with the demands of my work and family, and could run around with my kids until they asked me to stop! Any activity from then on was no problem.

Not only was there a definite increase in my physical flexibility and stamina, but I was also amazed at how wonderful I felt mentally. For the first time, I realized what Dr. Howard Murphy had implied with his statement, "It is impossible to walk rapidly and be unhappy." My attitude, confidence, and thinking potential reached new peaks. The feeling of well-being grew within me, and my need to continue with this experiment kept me on my toes (literally)! It did not stop there; as the weather changed to cold and rain, my determination to continue this positive effect led me to invest in a mini indoor gym! As if that wasn't enough, I got involved in acquiring knowledge and experience of all the possible beneficial exercises.

It is worthwhile to experiment with permutations and combinations until the schedule seems to be the most cost effective for each individual. In the meantime, keeping some simple, yet often overlooked, practical pointers in mind can go a long way in easing the experience.

The Environment

As you may have noted, what prompted me into this discovery was the association of physical activity with a friendly encounter. That was my motivation. As I walked and conversed with my well-wishing friend, I was actually enjoying the outing. The natural surroundings only enhanced the pleasurable experience. When I work out indoors on non-weather-permissible days, I use music or a TV show to keep me entertained. As a result, I am actually enjoying the time during which I am building my stamina. If you view exercising as a lackluster, compulsory activity, it will probably be depressing for you to get into it. So find a compatible and pleasant exercise buddy or invest in a treadmill to be placed near a music system or television and look forward to this fun and entertaining time of the day! (Time it with a comedy show and you will feel doubly refreshed, both physically and mentally.) Make sure you have some fresh air to join the party, and keep the temperature neither too hot nor too cold!

Proper Attire

Loose cotton clothing with well-fitting underclothes allows an easy workout and soaks up the sweat to allow comfortable physical exertion. Well-fitting, cushioned shoes with thick, soft cotton socks that prevent blistering and act as shock absorbers for the joints will ensure the longevity of this experience.

Meals and Fluids

It is probably not a good idea to work out an hour before or after a heavy meal. A light carbohydrate snack or a glass of juice twenty to thirty minutes before a workout will help prevent the faint feeling due to hypoglycemia (low blood sugar) that could occur if a meal was eaten more than three hours prior. Drinking plenty of fluids (ideally plain water that is not too cold; add electrolytes if intensive workout) helps replenish water lost from sweating and also helps wash out metabolites from the exercising muscles. One of these substances that can build up with intense exercising is Substance P, which causes the sensation of pain. Drinking an adequate amount of fluids ensures these metabolites are washed away easily, and therefore may help alleviate any painful sensation.

Chapter 28

Benefits of Exercising

According to the 2005 American Medical Association special release[36] *"the leading causes of death in 2000 were tobacco (435,000 deaths; 18.1% of total US deaths), poor diet and physical inactivity (400000 deaths; 16.6%), and alcohol consumption (85000 deaths; 3.5%)… However, poor diet and physical inactivity may soon overtake tobacco as the leading cause of death."*

It is therefore of immense importance that we fully recognize and utilize the advantages provided by exercising.

The benefits of regular physical exercising are too numerous to list. The following are some important ones worth discussing.

- Increases physical endurance

- Expends calories and helps regulate weight

- Lowers the incidence of coronary heart disease, high blood pressure, and strokes

- Alleviates the incidence and reduces severity of diabetes

- Might reduce risk of cancers, such as breast cancer

- Potentially helps improve mood disorders and depression

---

[36] URL- http://www.csdp.org/research/1238.pdf.

Exercising and Calories

Although the mainstay of any weight-loss program should be diet control, exercises do help in expending calories, thereby mobilizing fat. It also helps by raising the metabolic rate and therefore increasing calorie use. The amount of calories burned tends to be proportional to the intensity of the workout schedule. This is often referred to as the "activity factor." It is multiplied by the resting energy expenditure (REE), or basal energy expended by an individual during rest, to calculate the amount of energy spent performing an activity over a given time. An example of such calculations is given ahead.

Calories Expended in Exercising

Activity Factor	Activity	Calories Expended*
1 to 2 X REE$^\phi$	Standing activities Typing Painting Cooking	100-200 Cal/hr
2 to 3 X REE	Walking at 3 mph Golf Table tennis House cleaning	200-300 Cal/hr
5 X REE	Walking at 4 mph Cycling, Tennis Skiing Fast Dancing	400-600 Cal/hr
7 X REE	Football Basketball Climbing Heavy manual digging	600-700 Cal/hr

*Altered by the intensity, body, and lean weight of an individual
$^\phi$REE = resting energy expenditure

Other Benefits

In addition to increasing physical endurance and expending calories, regular exercising has been shown to lower the incidence of coronary heart disease and strokes. Some observational studies have hinted at a lower incidence of some form of malignancies, such as breast cancer, although direct association is still lacking. Interestingly, it may help in mood disorders as well, probably as a result of endorphins released in the body.

The Scientific Basis

One may wonder how an effort as simple as these physical exercises can have such widespread, beneficial effects. It is easy to understand the aspect of improved physical performance and stamina, since the muscle fibers are essentially stimulated to their optimum growth and activity potential with repeated practice. Interestingly, there are many case studies that associate routine exercises with longevity. This effect is possibly due to an increase in the heart's capacity to endure activity in an individual and the development of supportive circulation in the heart helping with the prevention of heart attacks. It probably has a more important although indirect effect of promoting weight loss and thereby lowering blood pressure.

The effects of exercising on creating a positive attitude, mood, and positive behaviors may be due to an increase in neurochemicals called endorphins being released in the body. Endorphins act on hippocampal regions of the brain, causing a feeling of happiness and decreasing pain perception. More recently, some studies have even shown a positive correlation of exercising with the reduced incidence of certain cancers, although this is debatable. If true, the exact mechanism by which this occurs is unknown.

There are just too many benefits to ignore this vital adjunct to our well-being, so let's get going (literally). You are already an ace if you are reading this book while running comfortably on a treadmill! Good luck and hope to see you on a marathon someday!

Chapter 29

How Much, How Often?

This is dependent upon the individual. Any amount of exercise is better than none. A minimum of twenty minutes three times a week has been shown to have beneficial health effects. According to the American Heart Association, the introduction of a dynamic exercise program of moderate intensity for thirty to sixty minutes three to six times a week improves the cardiovascular health of an individual. *However, before scheduling any degree of physical exertion in the form of structured exercises, it is imperative to get a complete checkup and clearance from your physician.*

For individuals who are starting exercise for the first time, it is recommended that they start slow and anticipate some muscle aches after the first few workouts as the muscles, which have not been used previously, are spurred into action. Plenty of fluids and an analgesic may help relieve these initial symptoms. For those with any known health care concerns and for those above fifty years of age, consultation with medical personnel prior to engaging in these activities is mandatory.

What About Intensity?

Dynamic, moderate-intensity exercise on a regular basis has been clearly shown to help lower the incidence of heart attacks, high blood pressure, and stroke. To define this, the concept of target heart rate was developed. I personally believe that exercising should be enjoyable and comfortable to the body. There is enough data to suggest that overexertion may, in fact, be harmful.

Athletes who perform excessive and strenuous exercises are more likely to have physiological and pathological disadvantages. Menstrual dysfunction, premature joint changes, and the predisposition to sudden heart attacks have all been associated with excessive physical exertion over long periods of time.

Many physical trainers and even machines are tuned to help an individual reach his or her target heart rate. The target heart rate[37] is 50 to 80 percent of the maximum possible heart rate for an individual and is a function of his or her age. This is usually thought to be around 50 percent to 80 percent of the maximum cardiac output.

Cardiac output is a function of heart rate and heart contractility, and it can be calculated by equations. One can get a rough idea by using the following formula:

Target heart rate =   (220 - Age) × 0.7

This may be an acceptable means if one uses pulse monitors or the palpation method (counting the pulse at the wrist for six seconds and multiplying it by ten). I prefer to exercise to my maximum level of comfort, which is usually shown by breaking out into a nice sweat without shaking up my body or having to stop with a pounding heart.

As we advance in our experience with exercising, we see that more and more can be done with the same feeling of comfort. In essence, slow and steady is much more likely to achieve desirable results than pushing the body to uncomfortable limits and quitting in disgust.

Another important fact that should be honored involves the adaptation process that our body deserves. In order not to perceive physical exercising as a stressful or painful experience, we need to gradually increase the intensity with warm-up exercises. These are

---

[37] URL- http://www.americanheart.org/presenter.jhtml?identifier=4736

low-impact and slower speed exertions that take place over a few minutes and prepare the body for a more aggressive exercising schedule. Similarly, at the completion of a workout, it is useful to perform some relaxing exercises before completely stopping; this is often alluded to as the *cool-down phase.*

Chapter 29

Types of Workout

Aerobic Exercises

"Walking is man's best medicine."
~Hippocrates, Greek physician (460-377 B.C.)

Walking, running, swimming, biking, etc. are all forms of exercises that tend to increase the cardiac output of an individual. Without increasing tension in a particular muscle, they induce an increased demand on the cardiovascular system due to the heightened activity of the person exercising. These exercises are also called isotonic (the tension on the muscles remains the same). Exertion of this kind increases the stamina of an individual so that the heart is able to do more work more comfortably with increasing practice.

There are lots of activities that we encounter in our daily lives that provide us with opportunities to do these exercises. For example, there were some days on which I had to go to four different hospitals to see my patients. The intensive care units in these hospitals were located on different floors—the third, fourth, and seventh. By the time I parked my car, walked to the hospital, climbed up the stairs (I hardly ever take the elevators any more), did my consultation, and headed back (and did the same with all the other hospitals), I was practically done with a good deal of my aerobic exercise needs of the day! Many people make healthy choices such as these in life to optimize time, efficiency, and—most importantly—health.

Another pleasurable form of aerobic workout is dancing. While the music rocks the soul, the lyrics elevate the psyche, and dancing charges up the body. What a wonderful way to get a total health experience!

One of the most pleasurable forms of exercising for me has become playing tag with my kids. By doing this, the whole family can have fun, increase their bonding, and work their hearts to increase capacity!

For those with joint diseases, it is most profitable to consider swimming exercises. Swimming allows a complete workout without building friction in the joints. Since the body is without the effect of gravity and therefore weightless in water, the bones and joints are not stressed.

Strengthening and Toning Exercises

While the aerobic exercises are aimed at working the whole body without building specific muscle power, toning exercises keep the body in a fixed position (isometric) and increase tension on groups of muscles. The intent here is to individually develop certain muscular entities so that higher forces may be generated as the muscle develops under repeated stimulus.

Using machines or weights, the muscles of the body are exercised individually or in groups to develop power. The number of times that the muscle is stimulated is measured in *reps*, and the duration one holds the muscle in its contracted state is *count time*. So, let's say you want to exercise your biceps (muscles located in the front of your upper arms). You could lift a weight that is just under the limits of being intolerable and you would bend your arm repeatedly for a total of, say, ten times (or reps), each time holding it in that position for a few seconds. Recently, physical trainers have discovered that fewer but slower reps are more apt to build a muscle group better. So instead of doing fifteen reps for seven seconds each time, it may be more effective to do ten reps for fourteen seconds each time. Regardless of whether you use the machine or free weights or do more or fewer reps, it is essential to do some form of muscle-stimulating exercise.

This form of exercise can be simply achieved by selecting weights (available in most general stores) that cause a tingling or burning sensation in the muscles when that weight is lifted, or by doing floor exercises. This is usually a weight that is just under the limits of tolerance. Different weights may be needed for different muscle groups, and varying actions will stimulate different muscle groups. For example, the upper extremity may be strengthened by lifting weights forward then upward or sideways then upwards. If you have access to a gym facility, practically every muscle group can be stimulated by working on the various machines!

The benefits of these toning exercises are increased muscular size, capacity, and endurance, which result in greater physical power. As we age, there is increased laxity of tissues, and not uncommonly, we see those sagging skins over a diminishing muscle mass. Since muscle is mainly protein, an increase in muscle mass helps replace fat under the skin. The body feels firmer, toned up, and solid. Strengthening and toning muscle-building exercises are meant to build muscle to its full potential, replace protein for fat, and allow an increased caloric requirement for the body.

Some women fear that if they indulge in these exercises, they will become manly in their appearance. This is probably not true, since the muscle mass in a woman is much less than a man's, even at peak development.

Stretching Exercises

In addition to building your cardiac reserve and strengthening and toning your body, it is worthwhile to stretch the tightening muscles, ligaments, and connective tissue to allow flexibility in the body. I have also found it a great way to release physical and mental stress.

Simple exercises include the following:

1. Bending forward and attempting to touch the toes with the fingers

2. Bending sideways with the hands on the hips.

3. Lying on your stomach and raising your head and upper body while being supported by the hands on the floor.

4. Lying on the stomach and holding the toes with your hand and raising the arms and feet.

5. Lying on the back and raising your arms and feet in the air as if doing cycling motions.

Yoga, an ancient form of disciplined control of body and mind, was first introduced thousands of years ago by a saint named Patanjali in India. In its original description, there were eight aspects of the practice that were undertaken to unite the body and mind with the soul and eventually with the supreme power (The word *Yog* means *to unite or link*). Subsequently, one of the eight aspects, *asana* (meaning posture), was elaborated by Yogi Swatmarama in the fifteenth century in India under the name of *Hatha* Yoga. This is what is commonly practiced in yoga classes in most of the world. It has some fascinating postures for promoting a flexible state, and it has been credited with many health benefits. It consists of attaining and maintaining various postures aimed mainly at stretching ligaments for flexibility and preventing joint diseases and also at strengthening groups of muscles that support the skeletal system of an individual.

Some remarkable forms of breathing exercises called *Pranayam* were also defined and presented by Saint Patanjali. These fascinating yet simple exercises served to keep the Yogis disease free, and they combined them with energizing meditation to achieve mental concentration, clarity, insight, and tranquility.[38]

---

[38]See the author's upcoming book, *Breath for Life: A Yogi's secret to health and Vitality*, for more details.

Chapter 30

Exercising Schedule

I strongly feel that each of the above forms of exercise (aerobic, strengthening, and stretching) should be included in an individual's workout schedule. Extremists in the field of physical training will promote just one form (either aerobics or weight training or stretching), but sooner or later the pendulum will swing in the other direction. If one objectively and scientifically analyzes these forms, one can understand why each of them should be a part of the exercising schedule.

How much each form should contribute depends on your age (older people need more aerobics) and your needs (body builders tend to use more strengthening and toning exercises). I, for example, spend about 60 percent of my time on aerobic exercises (four days in a week, thirty minutes each session), 20 percent on strengthening and toning, and 20 percent on stretching exercises (two days a week—twenty minutes of weight training and twenty minutes of stretching). You may want to take a session or two with a physical trainer at any exercise facility to get some ideas.

Regardless of what you eventually decide on, let me give you a few words of caution from experience:

- Do not get discouraged if you feel achy or tired in the first few days of your effort toward an active life (ensure first that you do not have any medical condition limiting your physical activity). The world experts on health issues will give their hearty approval because this is the most important step you are taking in your life. Continue with dedication and you will see the light at the end of tunnel. This should help you with your determination.

- Try to combine working out with a pleasurable event, such as walking with a friend, watching your favorite show, listening to enjoyable music, reading a book while on the treadmill or the stationery bike, etc. Feeling gloomy with weather blues? Go walking in a lively and well-lit mall (without your wallet)! Kids driving you crazy? Take them outdoors and start chasing them! This should keep you motivated.

- Exercise in moderation and on a regular basis. Excessive working out can be unhealthy for your joints and even the heart. Sporadic exercising does not have the same impact that regular exercising does. Even on vacation, find the time to be physically active. Having a workout schedule of four or five out of seven days allows you to make up for the days that you are just not able to get to it.

- In addition to paying close attention to the physical environment and personal attire and fluid needs, it is essential to give consideration to providing the body with adequate amounts of oxygen. This can be ensured by giving due attention to breathing and getting as much fresh air as possible (weather permitting!)

Got no time?

Those of us who have families, especially the ladies, will usually say, " I would love to, but I really don't have the time." How do I know? I have been there! So how do you find the time? My best friend often says, "You never have the time; you have to find the time!" So here are some simple suggestions that will get you going:

- As you read the section on time and space management and implement the suggestions, you will find those hidden time pockets that can be put to use for this important routine.

- If you have small kids who just will not let you be alone, you may alternate with your spouse or a friend or have the kids watch educational videos while you get in shape. (Our son learned his alphabets that way!)

- In case you have a YMCA or other such facility close by, it is worthwhile to enroll in it. Eating out one time less than the usual monthly number can easily make up for the monthly payment! While the kids have fun with their age-appropriate activities, you can enjoy the needful things.

- In case time constraints prevent driving to and from the facility, just create some space in front of the TV and get going. Initially, you may do your aerobics by jogging on the spot while you watch your favorite show or dancing in frenzy to an upbeat song. Stretching exercises are easy to do without equipment, and you may only need some weights (depending on your strength you will need a weight that produces a burning sensation in the muscles) for the strengthening and toning exercises. Probably the next birthday or anniversary gift can be a treadmill, a bike, or a complete, body-toning CardioGlide˚!

Rejuvenating Rest

Chapter 31

Restful Rest

"Sleep is the best meditation."
~Dalai Lama,

It is paradoxical to be discussing rest after energizing ourselves with physical exertion. But, indeed, these two aspects of health are like the two sides of a coin. Allowing the body and mind to undertake adequate rest enables the body to recover from the physical and mental strains of daily challenges. Probably no other form of rest is as complete in this regard as sleep, an event which helps an individual to physically repair tissues, clear the mind, and essentially recharge the system for new challenges.

In 2002, the National Annual Sleep Survey recognized that as many as 40 percent of young adults felt daytime sleepiness interfering with their functioning and increasing chances of accidents. Inadequate nighttime sleep and chronic sleep deprivation has been linked to health disorders like obesity and diabetes.[39]

Sleep

It is a recognized fact that sleep, as a period of compulsory rest, has the blessings and complete support of nature. The darkness and cool

---

[39] URL- http://www.nhlbi.nih.gov/health/prof/sleep/res_plan/section4/section4.html

that night brings with it is intended for us creatures to suspend our activities and lie down to enjoy the peaceful world of sleep. In fact, the body itself has the lowest concentration of the activity hormone called cortisol during this time. As an individual awakens, this hormone increases, and this cyclical change is what is referred to as the circadian rhythm.

During sleep, many changes vital to rejuvenation of the body and mind occur. The body functions are brought to their lowest states of metabolic activity; hence, there is conservation of energy. The caloric requirement to support this state is also at its minimum, which is referred to by scientists as the basal metabolic state. In this restful state, the body is able to expend more of its energy toward the repair of cells and tissues and the healing of its damaged systems. In a growing child, the maximum increase in the size of cells and tissues tends to occur at this time. This is due to a surge of a hormone called growth hormone from the pituitary gland, which is located in the midbrain. Growth hormone has the unique quality of building protein and other elements for cell growth and repair.

Sleep is also the only time (other than a coma!) when there is suspension of all active, conscious thought processes. This allows the brain to settle into a quieter pace of neuronal activity. However, this period of rest is not completely devoid of brain function, as baseline neuroelectric discharges are recorded even during sleep. Also, there is a period of sleep designated as REM (rapid eye movement) sleep, in which a person has increased brain activity. This period of sleep is associated with dreaming. Approximately 25 percent of the sleep duration is spent in this state, and it occurs about every ninety to one hundred minutes for increasing durations. This is in contrast to non-REM sleep, during which an individual has a quiet and diminished neuronal functioning. This period tends to occur before the period of REM sleep and after a period of light sleep. Therefore, a person is more likely to dream if he or she sleeps for a longer time.

The activity of the brain, as measured by electroencephalography, shows that neuronal discharges change with sleep stages. In the awake, alert, and actively thinking state, the brain emits low-amplitude, high-frequency electrical discharges that are called beta waves (fifteen to forty cycles per second). On attempting to sleep our brain waves become deeper, i.e. higher amplitude, and less frequent. These waves are called alpha waves (nine to fourteen cycles per second). Further deepening and reduction in frequency of waves occurs as we slip into a sleepy state with the onset of theta waves (five to eight cycles per second). These waves are also seen in daydreaming and during dreams in the sleep cycle. When deep, restful sleep is reached, our brains experience delta waves, the deepest and slowest waves of the sleep cycle (1.5 to 4 cycles per second).

Why Do We Sleep?

What constitutes this period of mental and physical tranquility is a mystery. Various brain centers, such as the reticular system, the thalamus, and neurotransmitters; such as Serotonin and others; have been implicated. Irrespective of the mechanism, there is no denying that rhythmic occurrence of this event is crucial to the well-being of an individual. Humans with sleep deprivation are noted to have increased periods of inattention, lack of focus, difficulty in retrieving information, and poor judgment. In specifically diminishing REM sleep over a prolonged period, detrimental effects on long-term memory were observed.

> *"A good laugh and a long sleep are the best cures in the doctor's book".*
> ~Irish Proverb

How much sleep a person needs is dependant upon the age and personal characteristics of an individual. A newborn sleeps sixteen to twenty out of twenty-four hours because it is in a period of rapid growth. On the other hand, an adult will feel refreshed after six to eight hours of peaceful sleep. With increasing age, most people report shorter durations of sleep and increased awakenings. The quality of sleep is as important as the duration. A shorter sleep without frequent awakenings and agitations is probably more beneficial than a long period of disrupted and restless sleep. In a study conducted in Australia and published in *Pediatrics*,[40] researchers confirmed poor general health and psychological distress in parents whose infants and preschoolers had sleep problems.

Disorders of sleep include sleepwalking and night terrors (night terrors occur almost exclusively in children). Adults may report frequent awakenings or shortened sleep due either to the inability to fall sleep or early rising—a condition also referred to as insomnia. On the other hand, some obese people may report frequent napping during the daytime due to severe snoring and respiratory pauses at night—a condition called sleep apnea. Most of these conditions need medical attention, although insomnia—the commonest of sleep disorders—is often a result of some other problem that may be transient, such as anxiety, depression, or situational stress. In the latter case, applying simple techniques to optimize sleep can help when used in conjunction with other important suggestions in this book—stress relief, regular exercising, and meditation in particular.

---

[40] Martin J., H. Hiscock, P. Hardy, B. Davey, and M. Wake. Adverse associations of infant and child sleep problems and parent health: an Australian population study. *Pediatrics.* 2007 May; 119(5): 947-55

Chapter 32

Optimizing Sleep

Everyone is not fortunate enough to fall asleep as soon as he or she lies down, nor are some lucky to get a refreshing, uninterrupted rest. And even an otherwise good sleeper may not be able to enjoy a restful night due to external or internal disturbances, be they physical or mental. There are certain steps one can take to enhance this blissful experience:

1. Sleep Timing

It is probably in the best interest of all concerned, whether children or adults, to maintain a routine in terms of the time for rest. As previously mentioned, the circadian rhythm of the body is set in such a way that neuroendocrinal changes in the body occur during resting times to allow a person to reduce his or her physical and mental activities. These get incorporated into an internal body clock, which helps maintain these changes rhythmically to keep in tune with different demands of day and night. If these limits are not respected, the body is bound to become imbalanced and unable to follow its internal cues and needs. It is indeed true when people say they cannot go to sleep easily when it is past their bedtime! A perfect example of this imbalance is the jet lag that people experience when traveling to a completely different time zone. Similarly, people who work in shifts with changing schedules will testify to this idiosyncrasy. So, unless it is absolutely out of your control, respect the timing!

2. Physical Environment

Approximately half an hour before bedtime, start turning off or dimming the household lights. The bedroom light should be dimmed, the TV should be turned off, and no work or stimulating reading should be undertaken in bed. Light or pleasurable reading, on the other hand, may be helpful. It is worthwhile to lower the temperature slightly below the "just-comfortable" zone to encourage inactivity and the desire to seek covers. Needless to say, the bed should be comfortable and the sheets should be of soft, absorbent quality (high linen content). Attention to the quality of the mattress and the support and comfort provided by the pillow will add to the restfulness of the sleep. In case you plan to sleep beyond sunrise, it may serve you well to have room-darkening blinds installed. (I use duette honeycomb blinds that come from Hunter Douglas!)

3. Meals and Liquids

The last heavy meal should be eaten at least an hour or two before bedtime. A time longer than that may result in stomach emptying and distraction due to hunger in some. Avoid spicy food if you have problems with falling asleep. Caffeine (coffee, strong tea, chocolate) or other stimulants should be avoided for at least four to six hours before sleep due to their awakening effect. I usually find that consuming a milk item such as yogurt or milk and cereal before bedtime is extremely conducive to promoting sleep. It has, in fact, been suggested that certain amino acids and elements in the combination of milk and cereal (such as tryptophan and calcium) may be responsible for this action due to the enhanced production of some specific neurotransmitters. In addition to attention to meal types and timings, it helps to avoid drinking fluids close to bedtime. Avoiding liquids at least two hours before the sleep time will help you to avoid unnecessary awakenings to go to the restroom, which would take away from your rest!

4. Physical Activity

Although most individuals are able to find time only in the evening to indulge in a structured physical activity, doing this too close to bedtime may be counterproductive. The body gets into a hypermetabolic state, causing it to release excitatory neurochemicals, which may prevent easy transition into a restful state. Therefore, performing such activities at least two to three hours (or earlier) before bedtime may be ideal. Strolls after dinner in a relaxed leisurely manner do not have the same effect and may actually help some people fall asleep.

5. Stress Relievers

Anxiety and distress are a sure way to lose sleep. Forget about being in bed; you might as well watch a funny movie! In case this is a major concern, referring to the suggestions in the section on stress management should provide some relief. For those of us who have bursts of ideas, realizations of unattended chores, or activities needing attention the following day, I highly recommend keeping some paper and a pencil next to the bed. As these thoughts strike you and disturb the slumber mood, simply write them down and make a habit of looking at them the first thing in the morning. Often, such thoughts create a mental stir because of the fear that one may not remember them the next day, which is addressed in this manner. In addition to using these general ways of relieving stress, I personally find taking a five- to seven-minute warm shower extremely helpful in falling into a quiet and peaceful sleep quickly. Also, during the last minute in the shower, try massaging all over using oil with sandalwood and lemongrass extracts (this should be occasional and with a small amount of oil to avoid absorption). As the aroma of this magical fragrance distracts the senses, it lulls an overactive brain to a zombie-like state, and pretty soon it is zzzzzzzzz time!

6. Tranquilizers

Medications directed specifically at inducing sleep should not be taken without medical consultation. These are often habit-forming substances that enhance a distorted sleep and have rebound effects, meaning that an individual may have either diminished or restless and unphysiological sleep cycles when their use is discontinued. In addition, cognizant mental activity may be impaired with some of these drugs. Both prescription (mainly bezodiazepines) and-over-the counter (mainly antihistamines) drugs can cause the above-mentioned problems. However, there may be justification for these in acute, stressful situations that are beyond personal control. The only time I would recommend these is if you have a big event the next day (such as your daughter's wedding!) and you will not be able to sleep due to intense excitement or anxiety, Here again it is important that you not be in a situation where you have to perform or be expected to remember issues the next day, as in an examination. Another example of the need for medical help may be to shorten the period of adjustment of jet lag in frequent business travelers. In these situations, the use of a hormone supplement called melatonin has been shown to be beneficial. Consultation with medical personnel before using these medications is recommended.

7. Natural Herbs

Nutritional stores provide sleep supplements made out of natural herbs that seem to work well for some people. I am not in a position to make recommendations regarding them, since the exact ingredients their side effects have not been not fully studied. I have occasionally used decaffeinated green tea for a soothing effect. Interestingly, I have found that chewing two 500 mg tablets of calcium (Tums*) or taking a calcium magnesium supplement seems to put me back to sleep easily when I am woken by a child in the middle of night. Again, milk and cereal seem to have the same effect on me when I have to interrupt my sleep for friends or family.

Chapter 32

Other Ways to Relax

One of the most pleasurable, relaxing moments in our family is watching a funny movie with the family while lying down and cuddling in a blanket. Some people can afford the luxury of short siestas in the daytime. Enjoyable, restful activities with friends can similarly have the desired effect.

Afternoon naps may be refreshing, but they are not advisable if night sleep is a concern. If, on the other hand, one is feeling extremely tired, it is counterproductive to postpone resting until late. Sometimes it is not a bad idea to take a short nap in the day if one is anticipating a late night due to an unavoidable social event. Naps completed before 2:00 p.m. are less likely to interfere with night rest.

A body massage with calming and sedative oils, such as eucalyptus, lemongrass, sandalwood etc., may be equally rewarding. A warm bath with aromatherapy can have a relaxing effect. Studies in animals have revealed that the stimulation of skin by gentle stroking produces healing factors, which scientifically supports the benefits of massage.

Reading a light fiction novel in a relaxing posture can similarly rest both the body and mind. Watching a comedy show while your feet are in a warm-water foot massager may serve well as a short, restful break.

Ensuring a comfortable posture (back rested and upright, arms at a comfortable distance, neck straight) before starting any task will go a long way in preventing fatigue and avoiding cervical (neck) disc injuries in the long run. Due attention to the position of the legs and back in activities involving the lower limbs may well prevent subsequent back pain or knee and ankle injuries. For example, I noticed that during some months, my left knee would hurt. After paying close attention and discussing it with a friend, I realized that I was holding my left leg in an inward position that caused it to awkwardly twist at the knee during driving. This was probably because of the close proximity of my seat to the steering wheel, and so during the months in which I did consultations for the university (which involves a lot of driving around), I was feeling discomfort, and eventually pain. Correcting the position of my leg relieved me of that discomfort and pain.

Yoga, a form of stretching exercise, has been scientifically shown to decrease cortisol levels and alpha brain waves, both of which are associated with a stress-free physiological state.[41] Meditation, a peaceful mental state described since ancient times, has similarly been shown to be associated with quieter brain activity, which is associated with feelings of peace and bliss.

There are many occasions on which we find ourselves waiting for another person (you know about this if you have kids or are dating!) or an event. This was often very stressful for me, as I often had 110 tasks listed for each day! I soon saw these as wonderfully relaxing and leisurely moments once I started keeping a book that I wanted to read and some relaxing or inspiring music with me in my car at all times. If I had to wait in the car, I had no problems, as I would lock my car, recline the seat, put on the music, and enjoy myself while relaxing. On the other hand, if I had to wait in a building (as was the case with my kid's music class), I would read my favorite literature!

---

[41] Kamei T., Y. Toriumi, H. Kimura, S. Ohno, H. Kumano, and K. Kimura. Decrease in serum cortisol during yoga exercise is correlated with alpha wave activation. *Perceptual & Motor Skills.* 2000 Jun; 90(3 Pt 1): 1027-32.

Soul

"What dothit profit a man if he gains the whole world and loses his own soul?"
~Jesus of Nazareth

It is a unique privilege for humans that we have the highest mental faculties among all animals. These faculties are needed to recognize the presence of a compelling power that cannot be seen, but only felt—a hidden dimension of life that we refer to as soul or spirit.

What is a soul? What is its correlate? Why do we need its realization?

It is an all-pervading animating principle, an omnipresent phenomenon responsible for life and motion, the strength of immeasurable possibilities within us, and the principles that govern the balance of nature.

Might it be energy? Might it be light? Whatever it is, it is the difference between a living person and a lifeless body. To ignore this essential attribute of health is like leaving a candle unlit, thereby denying it the very reason it was brought to existence. An individual who understands his soul, honors its presence, and works toward uplifting it is like a candle that burns with a wonderful aroma, touching the lives of all who cross its path. Let's be just that and enlighten our lives with an internal sunshine, rainbow, and aromatic garden. The journey may be made easy by:

- Recognizing the supreme power

- Discovering and evolving self

- Existing in harmony by observing laws of nature

Supreme Power

Chapter 33

Recognizing the Supreme Power

"I want to know God's thoughts; the rest are details."
~Albert Einstein

Probably about fifteen billion years ago, some powers or forces created conditions that caused the universe to manifest. Almost five billion years ago, the solar system materialized, and just a few hundred thousand years ago, man appeared on earth. What was there to begin with? There must have been some energy or some force that brought into existence everything that is now extant. That power, which sustains the universe, cycles life in every living being, from the smallest single-celled organism to the most complicated and intelligent organism yet identified—man.

We may not be able to see this power with our limited senses, but neither can we see electric currents. And yet, with a flick of the switch, when the current lights up a bulb, we give multiple theories about how the current must travel, how it can be altered, what its composition might be, and how it can be used. People who have had enlightening experiences with the supreme power can give similar details, but people must experience this unique phenomenon for themselves. Just as the taste of honey cannot be described other than by saying it is sweet, the experience of feeling the supreme power cannot be described either.

Scientific studies have shown that people with strong faith do better during recovery than those without the benefit of such support in life.[42] A study examining the effect of a three-day spiritual retreat on the feeling of well-being and social performance in heart patients conducted by University of Wisconsin confirmed the positive effect of faith and hope on healthy outcome.

Many people from the art and literary background often wonder if individuals following in the field of science believe in God. Their perception is that the concept of God explains what science cannot. This is far from reality. Science is discovering nature, not disputing it. Science still marvels at what it discovers. There is no denying that the processes occurring naturally—the programming built into every living thing that tells it to first grow, then mature, then regress and eventually dissipate—are planned to perfection. And yet, how has that been put in place, and by what or whom, and why? Can there be any denying of the fact that there has to be a power that is unseen yet felt, unheard but vibrating, nowhere and still omnipresent, mystical yet effective? It is this force that I refer to as supreme power. If you prefer to call it God, so be it.

For those of us who are still unsure about such an entity, the following is worth contemplation. If we accept this concept, we only serve ourselves better. In the absence of such a belief, where do we hang our faith? From where do we derive hope? Yet, without faith and hope, how does one proceed in life as one faces challenges, disappointments, distress, disease, old age, and eventually, death? It is impossible to be contented and peaceful—the basic prerequisites for our well-being—despite many adversities in life. How do we feel relaxed and stress free unless we have faith that everything will turn out the way it should once we have done our best and that the momentum set by our correct actions will be carried forth by the powers of universe to bring desirable results to fruition? As you attend to your tasks and duties day after day, some mystical force will guide them into appropriate consequences, and if the results that we are aiming for and the results we achieve are different, there is a reason behind it.

---

[42]URL- http://www.foxnews.com/story/0,2933,207881,00.html

"All things bright and beautiful
All creatures great and small
All things wise and wonderful
The Lord God made them all"

~Cecil Frances Alexander

I am reminded of the time we (my spouse and I) were working at a health care foundation that provided care for the under-served population without concern for cost. Our jobs were under a contract that was renewed annually. Since we liked being at the same setup and felt good about helping out the needy, we planned to continue our medical career at that setup. One year, as our contract came up for renewal, we discussed some issues with the administration and formalized the contract. Surprisingly, the next day, the administrator dealing with my spouse's contract declared that he had decided to sign on another physician instead. The reason the administrator indulged in such an unethical behavior is still unclear to us, but we knew that this was not a trustworthy environment in which to be. Although it was a distressing situation to be in, with a family of five to feed and home mortgages to be paid, we kept our faith and I confided in my fellowship director at the university, who had been my past supervisor. Sure enough, he told me that they would love to have me back and that interestingly, one of the faculty members had decided to leave due to family reasons. A few days later, he called back to say that the there was a vacancy in the field my spouse worked in and that since they held my husband in high regard, it would be their privilege if he decided to join them. So here we were a few months after experiencing a setback in our employment arrangements, comfortably working for a prestigious university, enjoying the intellectual stimulus, growing in our scientific background as we indulged in research, and enhancing our scholarly activities as we taught medical students and residents. In retrospect, I can see why things turned out the way they did, because that was a better plan than one we could have envisioned!

Faith does not just serve as a default directory in which our dreams may be stored for subsequent retrieval; it is a much more powerful phenomenon that affects our behavior, our perception, our thinking, our emotions, and even our bodies. In fact, there is now scientific evidence supporting the beneficial effect of faith on healing. There is evidence that the immune systems of individuals experiencing this phenomenon are enhanced and that recovery from surgeries is faster in those with spiritual beliefs. Patients indulging in spiritual practices have better prognoses when recovering from heart attacks and strokes. Even studies looking at the effect of prayers performed by other people for sick individuals have reported better outcomes in the people who were prayed for as compared to those who did not have such benefit! Miraculous recovery from various forms of cancers has been reported in patients who have had determination and faith. One of the greatest and most respected women of all times, Mother Teresa, had this to say about the strength of faith:

"I do not pray for success, I ask for faithfulness."
~ Mother Teresa

Attaining a healthier lifestyle, giving up addictions, consistently indulging in beneficial practices, and having good social relations have been seen more frequently in people who believe in God. Even life expectancy is higher in these individuals.

One such experience that I would like to share with you involves a baby who was born with complete paralysis of her entire body. This was extensive and severe, to the degree that she had to be placed on a ventilator (breathing machine) and given milk via a feeding tube to survive. While she underwent extensive testing and multiple neonatal and neurological consultations all over America, her condition showed no improvement. Days, and then months, passed without any shadow of recovery. During the third month of her life, I was involved in the care of the infant as a training physician. What struck me most was that her mother would sit next to her bedside and read her prayers from their holy scriptures every day. This was despite the fact that the mother had to care for two other small children at home. She would find relatives or friends, or she would wait until her husband got home, but she would be at the hospital each day.

The tests came back inconclusive, so a definite diagnosis could not be established. In the meantime, despite close attention to posture and physical therapy, the child was having other problems from chronic immobility. The condition was discussed with the parents, and possible options were discussed. The mother was convinced that the child would become better, if not normal. The care continued, and indeed the baby started showing some external movements. Slowly and steadily, she made progress. She eventually came off the ventilator, started feeding without a tube, and began demonstrating purposeful movement. This child subsequently learned to stand and walk, and her amazing story was even aired on television.

Chapter 34

Meeting the Supreme Power

Well, if there is such a power that guides everything into an appropriate consequence, maintains balance in the universe, and allows the harmonious existence of all matters, can we not experience it sometime? Yes, we can. Pick up a baby and see the perfection with which it has been created. Visit a garden and witness the undeniable beauty of the flora, leaves, flowers, and trees. Feel the energy transcend within as you smell a flower, hug a tree, or simply lie down on the grass and hug the earth. Spend time with nature; sit in stillness along an ocean, a river, or mountains, or just watch a sunrise or sunset and feel the presence of the supreme power. Gaze at the moon, stars, and clouds as they move across the sky. Or just sit still and transcend into meditation and feel this power within yourself, because this supreme power is as much a part of you as anything else that it creates.

My own first encounter with this supreme power occurred when I was around the age of sixteen. Although I used to accompany my grandmother to hear a spiritual leader speak for an hour every week on Sunday mornings, I was unsure if I really believed in this power. My visits to the spiritual gatherings were initially prompted by a need to provide her with physical help due to her severe arthritis, but I do admit that I subsequently started enjoying the spiritual discussions. In addition, my parents often visited religious places and took us with them, and I remember as a small child often looking up to the sky and talking to what I perceived as God.

The experience, which I can vividly remember to this date, took place on a winter evening when some of my friends and I had gotten together to have lunch and see a movie at a downtown location.

When the fun ended and it was time to go home, it was starting to get dark. My parents had gone to a dinner at their friend's house, so I was expected to use public transportation. I knew that I had to board bus #520 or 500 headed south. As my friends left in a hurry and I realized the urgency of time, I proceeded in the direction that I thought should be the bus stop area. Well, clearly I was wrong, as I circled for about half an hour before realizing that I was lost. Now, I had been told that as a rule of thumb, one (especially a young girl) should never make it apparent that he or she is lost when visiting the downtown area. I thought that I might be able to find a phone booth and call home, but I realized that no one was going to be there until later. It suddenly dawned on me that it was time to panic. Beads of perspiration collected on my forehead despite the cold, and I found each cell in my body praying with complete sincerity. Just then, I made a right turn, which was contrary to my mental calculations. As I stood waiting to cross that road, the light changed and the oncoming traffic stopped. My heart danced with joy as I saw right there, in front of all the vehicles in the right lane, the very bus I needed to board—bus #520. I rushed toward it and pleadingly waved to the driver with such vigor that he let me get in the bus. As I sat down, my mind was blank. I just stared ahead, almost not believing what had just happened. And then, when I reflected upon this later, I realized this could not have all been due to coincidence or chance. Why did I make the turn that my mind was strongly opposing? Why did the traffic lights turn red just at that moment? Why did I look to the side? What gave me the presence of mind to gesture to the driver in a manner that made him feel empathetic? What made the driver allow me to enter the bus against traffic rules? In short, what guided me to safety? Or should I say who?

Can this energy be felt at will? My recent encounters with some amazing energy forces during meditation retreats that use scientifically formulated exercises (with the Monroe Institute, USA) have convinced me of the validity of the experiences written about by others (such as *Autobiography of a Yogi* by Pramahansa Yogananda). It is my firm opinion that those who believe and are ready to receive are granted the manifestation of their desires.

Chapter 35

The Role of Religion

"They who have steeped their soul in prayer can every
anguish calmly bear."
~Richard M. Milnes

Once we realize the presence of this power, we often wonder what to
do to stay in tune with it. Many prefer to refer it to as God and use
religion to guide them to further their realization. It probably serves
some other functions as well. It allows one to have a structured and
scheduled way of maintaining his or her proximity with the divine
force. By meeting in groups at religious places—whether these are
churches, temples, mosques, monasteries, or any other structural
unit—people are able to reinforce their beliefs.

But each religion, with its structural unit, scriptures, teachings,
customs, and traditions, is merely a path to the ultimate reality. It
serves no purpose whatsoever to engage in religious activities if
the end result is not to respect that divine power and its creation.
And that creation includes you and me. It includes our families, our
friends, our colleagues, and our neighbors. It includes all the other
living and nonliving things, including this earth and this universe.
One of the greatest scientists of the twentieth century appropriately
declared:

Science without religion is lame, religion without science is
blind
~Albert Einstein

My children used to question me about other religions and why or how they are different. I told each of them to go outside and pick a different side of the house. I then asked them to describe what it looked like. The person in the front of the house described a door, a couple of square-shaped windows, an arch, a light hanging from the ceiling, and a brick exterior. The person inspecting the side saw no doors, one window, and wooden siding. Similarly, the individual looking at the back gave a totally different description. Now, when I asked them to come into the house and look around, they realized that it was the same house that they had described so differently. Similarly, the core values of each religion are essentially the same. Each religion professes love for each other, respect for mankind, the control of anger, forgiveness, and help for the needy. So why argue which religion is better? It is more important to make ourselves better.

How can any religion that condemns another be helping us to become closer to the supreme power if it cannot let us get closer to each other first? How can we reach out for the unknown if we do not reach out for the known? How can we respect the power that we cannot see unless we respect that power's creation, which we can see? The groups that engage in violence, disruption, and creating hate and anger toward one another in the name of religion are merely hiding behind the mask of so-called religion for ulterior motives and personal power. In becoming fanatic about a religion, one should not lose sight of spirituality. Religion is a road to spirituality—union of the soul with the supreme power. One should not get lost on the road, but continue to strive for the destination—the supreme power.

> *"The first purpose of prayer is to know God"*
> ~Charles L. Allen

A closer look at the origin, teachings and goals of each religion brings us to the realization that they are more similar to each other than different. Christianity, one of the more recently developed religions (about 2000 years ago), was inspired by the life and teachings of

Jesus of Nazarath, and it interestingly shares some common traits with one of the world's oldest existing religions, Hinduism. Both discuss the trinity. In the Bible, the holy scripture of Christians, the trinity consists of The Father, The Son, and The Holy Spirit. In the Bhagavad Gita, the holy scripture of Hindus, the trinity consists of *Aum, Tat,* and *Sat.* In both of these religions, unconditional love and faith in God is considered of prime importance for salvation and liberation (the terms for love are *Agape* in the Bible and *Bhakti Yoga* in the Bhagavad Gita). This is not different from the *complete surrender* of Islam, which originated in the seventh century when it was revealed by Muhammad and written in the Koran. While the Ten Commandments of the New and Old Testaments in Christianity speak of the moral conduct of an individual, the Hindu religion teaches, through the Vedas and the Bhagavad Gita, the importance of dharma (dutiful obedience of responsibilities) and karma (rightful action). Considering that the first incarnation of Hinduism existed in verbal form over 4000 years ago, it is clear that truth and good virtues, which are promoted by different religions, transcend time.

The roots of Christianity in Judaism (which originated at least a thousand years before Christianity) connect those two closely, just as Buddhism, Jainism, and Sikhism are religions that have developed from the original teachings of Hinduism.

All these different religions seem to have originated as an attempt to overcome the prevailing suffering, power, greed, and incorrect applications of teachings at the times when they were founded. For example, around the fifth century B.C., the interpretation of the Vedas had led to undue importance on rituals to the point that wisdom, insight, and conduct were being lost. Buddha (Sidharta Guatama), born into a Hindu family, felt the need to detach, concentrate, and gain knowledge of the ultimate truth with wisdom and insight to attain liberation. Indeed, if one looks closely at the teachings of the Bhagvad Gita (Hindu religion), it seems that out of the paths towards *Moksha* (liberation) mentioned in it, there are the following: *Karma* (rightful action) *yoga, Jnan* (knowledge) *yoga,* and *Bhakti* (devotion) *yoga.* Buddha chose the path of knowledge and insight. The Four Noble Truths of Buddhism are based on principles of gaining knowledge and insight into the truth of suffering in life produced due to attachment to things and desires, and he stressed the need for mankind to strive for *Nirvana* (liberation, or freedom from suffering). He discussed The Eightfold Path of right speech, action, livelihood, effort, mindfulness, concentration, thoughts, and understanding as a template for rightful living.

In essence, all religions were developed as a need for man to realize that there is more to life than living like animals, merely pursuing sensual pleasures, and existing in material form. They teach that the higher intelligence of humans should allow them to live and conduct themselves in a manner that befits their higher evolution and is supportive of others and nature by incorporating virtues and values. And beyond that, they teach humans to seek freedom from fears and suffering by respecting, honoring, and loving the power that creates and sustains, thus allowing each of us to have faith and hope and an opportunity to live in peace.

In one of the inspiring lectures delivered at St. Louis University by Father Gray, a professor from Boston College, a person from the audience asked him in what light he saw and dealt with inter-religious communication and how he saw things differently now that he was older. The distinguished speaker paused for a moment, and in a very humble and sincere manner he replied, "Earlier I used to think when I met people of other religion that I have something that they don't. Now I feel that they probably have something that I don't." It cannot be said with more honesty and sincerity than that! I could see that this man had crossed the boundaries that man creates around himself to stifle his connections with the universe. He had broken the chains of interpretation that we force on our community. He is truly liberated and free to experience the presence of the divine power in all its manifestations. For as a distinguished former U.S. president said:

> "When I do good, I feel good. When I do bad, I feel bad. And that's my religion."
> ~Abraham Lincoln, U.S. president

Chapter 36

Reaching Out and Empowering

When we let go of our prejudices and our preconceived notions and become more attentive to our environment, only then do we awaken to the presence of the supreme power and its abundant energies. It awakens us to those limitless potentials within us.

The other day, as I was driving out of the hospital parking lot of a in my car, I saw an older man looking confused and worried as he searched for his car. I could empathize with him about the distress felt when one is lost (I've been there more than once!), especially because it was cold. Even though I realized that his ethnic background and religion were different, it did not dissuade me from reaching out to help. As I drove up to him and offered help in taking him around the five-level parking lot to locate his car, I could see a slight hesitation on his part. He was probably reluctant to inconvenience a physician, as we are always pressed for time. After a brief moment, he stepped in, thanking me for the offer. As we drove around, we realized that he had exited the building on the wrong floor and that his car was parked on the third level though he had been looking on the first. As he got out of my car, he folded his hands together and said, "Thank you very much." My soul filled up with a glowing light as I realized how our spirits had connected. I did not feel proud of what I did, and I will not even accept it as a helpful gesture; to me it was an event that connected me with this individual through the divine power.

It was an acknowledgement that the almighty uses his creation to help his creation. Now, I am not promoting helping out strangers and thereby helping people with criminal intent to find easy prey, but after assessing the genuineness of the situation and the probability of any harm being done, helping someone is a powerful lesson in experiencing spirituality.

Why do we feel happy and peaceful in similar encounters in which we have been of service to another individual? Scientifically, such experiences have been linked with the release of chemicals called endorphins within our bodies. This is responsible for a feeling of euphoria, ecstasy, or a feeling of peace and blissfulness. That is why it is easy to see why spiritual practices have helped people with mental disorders like depression and drug addiction.

Spirituality and Self-Evolution

"And above all things, never think that you're not good enough yourself. A man should never think that. My belief is that people will take you at your own reckoning."
~Anthony Trollope

In some Asian cultures, people greet each other by putting their hands together and bowing. The true meaning of this gesture is very deeply rooted. The palms of the hands symbolize the soul, while the five fingers symbolize the five senses of an individual. Through this gesture of putting the palms together, the gesturers acknowledge that despite their perceiving the world differently due to their distinct senses, their souls are connected because they belong to a universal spirit. And by bowing, they show respect to each other and the supreme power, of which they all are a part.

By believing in these powers within us, we can work toward raising ourselves to limitless potentials. As in the words of Søren Kierkegaard,

"It is very dangerous to go into eternity with possibilities which has oneself prevented from becoming realities. A possibility is a hint from God."

Spirituality and Death

"After your death you will be what you were before your birth."

~Arthur Schopenhauer

Death, to many of us, is an end to our physical form. However, death does not end life; it completes it. Death is clearly as much a reality as is the fact that we are born. No one can escape that event, and it truly is the only sure occurrence in life after birth! And yet it is the thing many of us are least prepared for. We may have insurance policies in place, wills locked up in safes, and guardians picked out for our children, but what are we going to be thinking about when we have to endure it? More difficult still, how do people cope with the death of a loved one? Spirituality is our only savior in these distressing moments.

I am reminded of a circumstance in which this was beautifully exemplified. An infant was born with a congenital defect that was incompatible with life and incurable. The family was aware of this due to an antenatal ultrasound. They had undergone extensive counseling and had good social support available at the time of their baby's birth. Yet the birth of the baby was a traumatic event for the family, and the mother was scared, and she struggled to hold the baby and emotionally struggled to keep the baby home. After the involvement of pastoral care, elderly family members, and counseling teams, there was a remarkable change in attitude and an acceptance of the situation. They named the baby after an angel and announced that the infant was a little angel visiting from heaven to bless them.

The family and friends loved and caressed the baby until its last breath, and they found themselves stronger from the experience.

When we have an unshaken faith in the divine power, we do not question that death is only an end to our earthly existence. We believe that we join our creator in spirit, and as per some religious beliefs, that we even return to earth in another life—a phenomenon referred to as *reincarnation*. Even people whose religious beliefs dispute this have encounters with this phenomenon, as is amply exemplified in the writings of Dr. Weiss, such as *Many Lives Many Masters*.

Regardless of what our faith leads us to believe, we do have the hope of existence in some form after death. This takes care of some our basic fears, including fear of the unknown and fear of extinction. Even we, struggling with disease, disability, disappointments, old age, and distress from any other challenge, need faith and hope to survive. Despite such adversities, if we believe in a higher power, life can be navigated using ease, peace, and calm. Once we have conceptualized the supreme power, visualized its potentials, entrusted our present and future to it, and realized that we are merely an extension of it, there is no unknown and no extinction. As in the words of a yogi named BKS Iyenger, "The finite joins the infinite and becomes infinite itself." With this belief, one realizes that life will be fine and that death is not a concern! Nothing can have a more powerful positive influence on our well-being.

Evolving Self

Chapter 37

Self-Awareness

"*I want, by understanding myself, to understand others.
I want to be all that I am capable of becoming...........
This all sounds very strenuous and serious. But now that I
have wrestled with it, it's no longer so. I feel happy -- deep
down. All is well.*"

~Katherine Mansfield

It will serve us well at this stage to put aside this book and suspend all other activities for just one minute after reading this paragraph. Either write down or visualize at least twenty people whom you feel very close to and think you know well. These may be from your workplace, family, circle of friends, or social groups that you participate in. From these, pick out your favorite individual whom you also are most knowledgeable about, and then read the next paragraph.

You have just gone down your memory path and selected an individual whom you have met, conversed with, spent time with, interacted with, and built a mental image of through introjections or projections. Essentially, you have become familiar with this person to an extent that you probably know his or her strengths and weaknesses, likes and dislikes, mood swings, and other aspects of their character. You are probably also aware as to what is most appealing and comforting to this person. Now, is this person you? Why not? Why is it that you know some people well—people whom you meet and interact with sometimes—and yet do not thoroughly know the person you are all the time—yourself!

Why do we need to know ourselves better than any of our acquaintances? Why should we try to seek ourselves, indulge in our own self-images, and explore our true beings? The answer is simple: Without self-awareness there can be no self-awakening, and without self-awakening, there can be no self-evolution. Unless we strive toward self-evolution, we will be struggling for the rest of our lives for a feeling of well-being at the mercy of other people and external objects. Our possessions, our social interactions, and the situations that we find ourselves in will dictate our emotional states. If you look at each of these items, you will realize that in a dependent state, we really do not have any control over any of them. A person who allows these things to influence and control him or her can never rise above internal struggles. The ways in which people treat us, the kinds of situations we have to face, and what our eventual materialistic achievements can be will always overwhelm us unless we take control of just one thing, and that is ourselves! Sir Oliver Holmes put it very well when he wrote, "What lies behind us and what lies before us are tiny matters to what lies within us."

Discovering Self

"*The worst loneliness is not to be comfortable with yourself.*"

~Williams James

The first thing an individual should with all honesty and commitment try to achieve is an understanding of oneself. Who are we? What is our mental makeup? How do we act and react? What characteristics do we display? Are these characteristics desirable or undesirable? What is our inherent nature? Are the qualities that make up our individuality the same that we would like others to show toward us? What is our role in this universe?

"One must know oneself. If this does not serve to discover truth, it at least serves as a rule of life and there is nothing better."

~Blaise Pascal

To start with, find a quiet place by yourself and reflect upon the day's events, observing yourself as an actor. For us to be able to know ourselves and objectively analyze the information, we need to enforce two simple rules. Firstly, detach your self from yourself. In other words, observe yourself from the eyes of another person—say, a bystander. Secondly, be nonjudgmental: do not praise or criticize, do not think positively or negatively, but just have a neutral attitude. Let all the observations just come and pass. In case some are particularly disturbing and keep recurring in your memory, write them down. As in the words of Paul Tillich, "The courage to be is the courage to accept oneself, in spite of being unacceptable."

As you advance in this stage of self-recognition and start getting comfortable with yourself, it may be worth venturing to the next level of self-analysis. This is often difficult and not always feasible, and it may be easier if you have a respectable soul mate. Among the people you know, be it your spouse, your close friend, or your sibling, there is often some person whom you completely trust and with whom you can freely discuss any issue. Evaluate whether this person can help you get more objective data on your being. If this is a particularly difficult proposition, it does not need to be embarked upon.

It is important that we not react to the information that is presented to us. This tends to occur if we forget that we are observing actions and feelings as a director, as an observer, and not as an actor or the doer. Some of our physiological processes, such as fast breathing, and the awareness of heart beating, can help us recognize that we may be reacting to the information that we are reflecting upon or becoming judgmental. With experience, we will be able to allow our minds to wander into events of the past that may have been repressed. This will permit us to free our minds of many resentful, fearful, depressing thoughts that we often carry buried in the unconscious mind, which deprives us of our energies, prevents us from keeping an open mind, and robs us of our full potentials. As we will see in the section on self-evolution, dealing with these repressed images will bring us to experience new heights in mental freedom, exquisite happiness, and ultimate peace.

"As soon as you trust yourself, you will know how to live."
~Johann von Goethe

Chapter 38

Self-Awakening

"The hell to be endured hereafter, of which theology tells, is no worse than the hell we make for ourselves in this world by habitually fashioning our characters in the wrong way."
~Williams James

Once you have realized "self" and become aware of the idiosyncrasies of your inherent nature, it is time to apply it to your present life. Self awareness has been referred to here as a process of retrospective (as it happened) analysis of being. Once this is accomplished, it would be prudent to introduce the concept of *self-awakening* as the application of the same principle prospectively (as it *is* happening). Essentially, it is a nonjudgmental analysis of how one is manifesting one's being in a situation, be it in the form of actions, perceptions, thoughts, feelings, or emotions. It is similar to making a video recording of an individual as events are occurring. In other words, it means being mentally awake and therefore knowledgeable about how we are conducting ourselves externally and allowing ourselves to be influenced internally by our physical and emotional environment.

Here is an example that may serve as a powerful tool in helping you to understand this better. Occasionally, I have witnessed an interesting situation develop in the waiting rooms of our medical clinic. A parent will be waiting with two or more of his or her children in the waiting room, and suddenly, for no apparent reason, one of them will start crying loudly. One child will start shouting at the other child, and a physical fight will occasionally ensue. The reactions of the parent are sometimes worth recording. They will show their disturbance visibly and start shouting themselves, often saying, "Don't shout! I said don't shout!" Then, if they are not able to control the situation, they will slap the child who is most likely to have caused the problem (usually the older one) and retort, "Don't hit the baby; do you understand?"

This is not intended to mock or belittle the conduct of poor parents who are harassed by the situation and their reflex reactions to rectify the imbalance and regain what they might perceive as dignity of some sort. I am sure all of us may have unknowingly acted similarly if put in their shoes. But let us analyze this objectively. Kids fighting and crying is as acceptable as a man working for a living! It is part of their job.

Letting a natural phenomenon bother you without understanding allows you to act irrationally, feel overwhelmed, and lose your balance. Shouting at them while telling them not to shout sends them the message, "You can shout when you are bigger or in power!" Slapping one of them reinforces that violence may be used to demonstrate authority and control over a situation. Onlookers can understand the kids' behavior because they are below the power of reasoning. The adults, however, displayed some concerning traits. In addition, they promoted unhealthy behavior in the children and probably earned some guilt for themselves.

If these parents had been practicing self-awareness and awakening, they would have realized the irrational reactions that were being generated within them, and they probably would have acted in a peaceful and more effective manner. This would have included removing the younger child from the reach of the older, discussing the reason for the child's behavior with them, and using consequences such as showing disapproval and maybe the withdrawal of some privileges, such as TV time, toys, or playtime with friends, to discourage the behavior. Or better still, they could have developed a positive reinforcement strategy to bring out the best behavior in their children.

One can see how we can prevent a disturbing, unsettling, and chaotic situation by simply observing ourselves closely and prospectively intervening with appropriate measures to allow our selves to manifest in a peaceful, unstressed, and comfortable manner. Regardless of the situation, we can stay in control and function with reasoning, insight, and effectiveness.

We will not know what to do in every eventuality, nor can we be knowledgeable about the technicalities of every situation, but if we allow our inner self to manifest without embarrassment, fear, or anger while being cognizant of our instincts, we are most likely to do our best. And that is essentially what self-awakening is.

> *"People seem not to see that their opinion of the world is also a confession of character."*
> ~Ralph Waldo Emerson

It Doesn't Stop There!

Why is this exercise of observing our thoughts and actions really a spiritual one rather a mental one? Because it fulfills the needs of our souls as it allows us the opportunity to develop our characters. Knowing that we have done our best in the circumstances in which we have been placed is the best soul food. In the words of Marion L. Burton, "From self alone expect applause." It is this applause that reverberates in our spirits, kindles our inner selves, and soothes our souls, granting us the unmatched feeling of well-being.

And yet, despite all the efforts and best intentions, we all have imperfections. William Sloane Coffin had a good perception of this when he reflected, "I am not okay, you're not okay—and that is okay." But the soul, once kindled in this way, craves higher grounds. Just like we look in the mirror every day and make appropriate amends in our appearances so that we can look better, once we start looking within ourselves we want to be better. Only when we have we acknowledged our imperfections can we strive toward improving upon them.

> *"Growth begins when we start to accept our weakness."*
> ~Jean Vanier

In other words, once we have reached a state of self-awakening we are now equipped to progress to self-evolution.

Chapter 39

Self-Evolution

"Alas, after a certain age, every man is responsible for his own face."

~Albert Camus

Probably the most pivotal and uplifting experience one can have is the realization that we are an integral part of nature and an extension of the supreme power. If we envision the supreme power as the sun and ourselves as rays, it is easy to see that the glow in our life is only possible when we are connected to the sun. All other living things are a part of that supreme power, just like us, and they are therefore connected to us.

It is an indescribable state of existence when the light fills our souls after we incorporate this wisdom within us and appreciate the presence of all components essential for unlimited potential, boundless energy, and priceless grace of the universe. Self-evolution is a state in which we empower ourselves by being our best selves.

Let me share a personal experience that I feel might enlighten you about such a phenomenon. My personal self-awareness and awakening brought to my attention the impatience that I would demonstrate toward my kids and spouse in times of stress. I could also analyze myself at work, where I repeatedly visualized myself as extremely well disciplined and personifying all the appropriate characteristics of a balanced individual. My practice as an intensivist often puts me in situations in which I am dealing with life-and-death scenarios and maintaining peacefulness and calmness as a team leader to help achieve positive results. In addition, it is probably unlikely that my co-workers would put up with any less-than-desirable behavior. However, when I started observing my lack of control regarding my temper toward my family, I found it extremely disturbing. How could I not want the most positive outcome for the people who mattered to me most? Should I not be paying close attention to the needs of my own family rather than reacting to imperfections and thereby creating more imperfections?

Self-evolution is indeed a difficult yet crucial step toward self-fulfillment. And yet, self-fulfillment is a prerequisite for a state of complete well-being. It is like the sugar in a cake recipe; without it, there is no taste. Despite being baked to perfection, the cake can never taste right if the sweetness is missing. Again, probably the most useful exercise in this process is understanding, analyzing, and correcting oneself by paying closer attention to the self. Keeping the company of evolved individuals in person or through books helps reinforce and firm up our conceptions. Indeed, we can conquer the world once we conquer ourselves. As in the words of the famous Roman author:

> *"Most powerful is he who has himself in his own power."*
> ~Lucius Annaeus.

Empowering ourselves by recognizing the blessings of the Supreme power and striving to exist in harmony with the extension of its creation we should evolve ourselves through respecting and reflecting the laws of nature.

The Laws of Nature

Chapter 40

In Harmony with Nature

"The rule of joy and the law of duty seem to me all one."
~Oliver Wendell Holmes

Every individual, community, association, organization, city, state, nation, and for that matter the entire world, is able to function in some form of balance by observing certain rules and regulations. In the absence of such principles, there is bound to be chaos, disruption, and no scope for any peace or progress. These rules and regulations that are man-made are usually available in some format and referred to as written laws. If an individual does not obey them, it is grounds for action against that person, and he or she is then responsible for attending to the consequences.

If man-made aggregations have used this method to allow smooth running, it stands to reason that this universe, which was created to perfection by the supreme power, uses the same type of rules? These are not written anywhere (unfortunately, like babies, nature does not come with written instructions!), but the intelligent mind can perceive them. It does not need to be told what is needed to maintain balance in this universe or what would happen if these laws were indeed broken. It is therefore for our own benefit that we fully recognize, understand, and apply to our lives these laws of nature. A sensitive and appreciative mind can relate to some of the most important ones, which I feel compelled to discuss here.

Each individual has his or her own perception of what is most conducive to harmonious existence. In my opinion the following are the most important aspects that need to be recognized, understood and integrated in our lives to allow a peaceful, blissful and healthy existence. The word *CIRCLES* sums up these elements, and symbolizes the ripple effect it has on the quality of our lives:

C Compassion

I Intent and Action

R Respect

C Creativity

L Love

E Enjoyment and Appreciation

S Service and Sincerity

Chapter 41

The Circle of Life: Compassion

"Do unto others as you would have them do unto you."
~Jesus of Nazareth

"What goes around comes around." "Treat others as you would like to be treated yourself." We have heard these kinds of statements so many times that we have probably never realized how powerful and universally encompassing the underlying, simple rule is. Try to visualize a community, an organization, or a nation in which people compassionately treat another person, expecting to be treated in a similar way. How smoothly, how effortlessly, how efficiently, and how peacefully would the system function?

The very circle of life is arranged in a manner that causes you to eventually become a part of the substance that you have been extracting from. A plant grows from a seed, and yet the seed comes from a plant. The plant draws upon the resources of the soil, and yet when its life is over, it returns to that same soil. While the soil provides for the need of the plant, the plant provides for the needs of the soil; both enrich each other, and both are dependent upon each other. What better cooperative existence can there be? You have to give back what you get to complete the circle of life.

"If we have no peace, it is because we have forgotten that we belong to each other".
~Mother Teresa

213

Then the same rule should apply prospectively, too; that is, in order to receive, one must give. How can one expect to receive if one does not give? We work hard at our jobs and receive rewards for that. We give fertilizer and water to a tree that bears flowers or fruits, and we reap the benefits of nature's beauty.

This does not only apply to materialistic possessions; it is as important, if not more so, to practice it in the behavior, actions, feelings, and emotions that we apply to others. If you treat your spouse with love and dignity, you will enjoy a happy relationship together. If you give time, attention, and care to your kids, you will have many reasons to be proud of them.

Allow your thoughts, words, and actions to be guided by honesty and you will find honesty smiling back. Treat others with love and you will receive love. Treat others with respect and you will be respected. On the other hand, show hate and hate will be returned to you. If we live with bitterness, then bitterness will stare back at us every day. Those who achieve by deceit and wrongdoing will meet deceit paying them back pretty soon. It really is as simple as that.

> *"If you want others to be happy, practice compassion. If you want to be happy, practice compassion. "*
> ~Dalai Lama

A few months ago, I had an interesting incident. I returned to my car in the parking lot after shopping at a department store. There standing next to my car was a young girl, and as I tried to get into my vehicle she approached me and gently said, "Excuse me!" I thought my open door was preventing her from moving so I closed my door and started the engine. She started knocking at the door, which surprised me somewhat. I opened my window, and she said in a very apologetic tone that she had hit the side of my van while she was reversing. Since she did not know whose van it was, she had waited in the parking lot to inform the driver, and she hoped that I was not going to be mad about it. Her honesty and sincerity completely amazed me, considering that this was coming from a teenager. I shook my head and said, "Not at all. What you have just done deserves the highest praise possible. Whether my insurance or yours picks up the bill is going to be immaterial, but the strength of character and values that you have shown are going to be your life achievement. The structural and minor fiscal damage that we may incur will be soon recovered, but the respect and self-esteem that you have earned, no one will ever be able to take away from you." I subsequently wrote her a reference letter highlighting the honesty, courage, responsibility, and sensitivity shown by her action.

How do we always remain cognizant of this rule so that we act with compassion and justice? A simple way is to practice empathy. Empathy means placing yourself in the other person's shoes and recognizing his or her thoughts, feelings, and emotions. This is much more involved than sympathy, which merely induces pity. Only by placing ourselves in the other person's position can we have the true perception of what it must be like to be the receiver. Then and only then can we give of our materialistic possessions, actions, and emotional support with any justification.

We are often in situations in which we are too hindered by our past negative experiences with an individual to apply empathy. Holding grudges and prejudices and allowing egotistic interpretations prevent us from keeping ourselves in balance and harmony with other souls. The one most enriching experience for the soul is probably practicing forgiveness. It leaves a joyous aroma that is soothing, uplifting, and majestic. How well it has been embodied in this beautiful quotation:

> *"Forgiveness is the scent that the rose leaves on the heel that crushes it."*
>
> ~Anonymous

Amazingly, as one starts to practice this law, the act of giving itself becomes a reward to the giver. As one relates oneself to the supreme, as one indulges in self-evolution, and as one extends his or her generosity to the other creations of the supreme, one realizes how much richer everyone has become. In this manner, people can start the journey in an upward spiral, lifting themselves up to the heights of boundless spiritual wealth that no one can rob them of.

Chapter 42

The Core of Existence: Intent and Action

"What can be added to the happiness of a man who is in health, out of debt, and has a clear conscience?"
~Adam Smith

Time and again we are in situations that disturb our inner harmony because of another person's intent or action. I am not referring here to misunderstandings and the like, but to clear acts of wrongdoing. If this individual is a person whom we trust and respect, it infiltrates deep into our conscious—and probably subconscious—thinking. The ripple effect is commonly obvious in our emotional reactions, attitudes, and behavior. No amount of explaining, sweet talk, or persuasion seems to lend a healing touch to the wounds that have so influenced our very existence. The repercussions are deep and widespread, and it is difficult to reverse the effects of wrongdoing.

This helps us realize how crucial it is to try to sincerely embody an honest intent and attempt the correct action.

Among all the virtues that an individual can display, probably the most noble and compelling is honesty. An honest intent and action needs no clarification and stands the test of time eternally.

"Honesty is the first chapter in the book of wisdom."
~Thomas Jefferson

The first task we should embark upon is to address our own intent in life. We need to explore within us our mission on earth, our role in the universe, and the actions desired of us in achieving our goals. It is easy then to put life and its existence in a mortal form in their true perspective. It would then become easy for us to plan for the year, month, week, and each day. In moments of stress or during misconceptions, it is not uncommon to lose our bearings. It may serve us well to have our actions be influenced by uplifting and nourishing quotations by great authors.

Action guided by honesty, wisdom, compassion, and contemplation will go much further than envisioned. Realizing that inaction is sometimes a better substitute than any form of inappropriate action is only possible when an individual applies these principles to reason with intent and action.

> *"Fate gives us the hand, and we play the cards."*
> ~Arthur Schopenhauer

Chapter 43

The Fundamental Approach: Respect

"Provision for others is a fundamental responsibility of human life."

~Woodrow Wilson

Respect is an expression of regard or consideration toward another individual. It is amazing how easily tasks get accomplished without friction, disgruntlement, and chaos once this fundamental approach is used. Also, a feeling of justice and tranquility prevails in all those participating in respecting one another.

Not uncommonly, we feel that we deserve more respect from our so-called subordinates, be they co-workers or tiny family members at home. But how many times do we analyze our own behavior toward them? How many times do we say "could you please get this done by this date" versus "I need this by this date"? Next time you call any organization, ask very politely with a "please" at the beginning of the sentence. Invariably, you will hear a very enthusiastic "sure" on the other side of the phone (unless the person on the other side has just been rebuffed!). Just by addressing another individual in an appropriate, respectful light, one is able to start a relationship on the right footing. This allows a peaceful and happy environment for all concerned, which relaxes the soul.

Respect; not only for another individuals, but also for other living things and our environments; allows us to be in harmony within our ecosystem. Whether it involves the plants or animals or physical environment, respecting our surroundings is an essential prerequisite for a harmonious existence.

And above all, respect for self is of prime importance. By allowing ourselves consideration, regard, and dignity we maintain our self-esteem. Self-esteem is like the backbone of our soul, because without self-esteem, we set ourselves up to be repeatedly hurt by others. Unless we consciously (and eventually unconsciously) practice this fundamental approach, our well-being will always be at the mercy of other people's behavior, feelings, and emotions.

> *"No one can make you feel inferior without your consent."*
> ~Eleanor Roosevelt

Chapter 44

The Uplifting Emotion: Love

"One word frees us of all the weight and pain of life. The word is love."

~Sophocles

An acclaimed Greek dramatist who lived about four hundred years before Christ knew the power of this one emotion—love. Psychologists talk about eight primary emotions that are comprehended by a human: joy, acceptance, fear, surprise, sadness, disgust, anger, and anticipation. When joy and acceptance are put together, the resultant emotion is love—a form of secondary emotion. And when joy and anticipation are blended, we get optimism. This helps us see that love is a blended emotion of two very comforting feelings within us: joy and acceptance.

Although love itself has been described by some as having the qualities of either passion, sensuality, friendship, logic, possessiveness, or selflessness, it is the last one that I refer to here. Also described as *agape*, this form of love is the purest and most uplifting emotion that an individual can experience. To the receiver, it is the most comforting and motivating feeling displayed.

And yet it is probably the most powerful emotion between two individuals. A person can be spurred to any action or inaction by this emotion. Let me bring to your attention a symbolic childhood story that highlights this phenomenon. You might recollect Aesop's story of the sun and the wind. For those who do not, this is how it goes:

"A man was walking down a country road with his hat and coat on. The wind [symbolizing criticism and harsh words] challenged the sun [symbolizing warmth and love] that it can blow away the man's coat. Sun accepted the challenge and watched as the wind hemmed and hawed to blow away the man's coat. Interestingly, the more the wind blew, the more the man held on to his belongings. Finally, the Sun asked for a few moments of trial. Sure enough, as soon as the Sun started shining brightly, the man took off his coat. Moral of the story, you can make someone do what is needed by being warm and kind, while criticism and harsh words only makes one rebel."

There are those among us who consider anger and force as strong motivating factors for compelling others into action and getting effective results. On the contrary, these are actually weapons of the weak-minded individual who is attempting to light the forest by using fire. What that person does not realize is that everything will eventually be destroyed.

> *We must interpret a bad temper as a sign of inferiority.*
> ~Alfred Adler

This brings us to some burning issues in our country. We seem to be chasing our tail while dealing with problems affecting our teenagers. Sex, violence, and drugs have slowly infiltrated our society, and we are unable to reverse the stronghold. We, as adult mentors, go from permissiveness to aggressiveness without any desirable results. At times when these growing minds need guidance, we are unavailable, and then when we are confronted by their inappropriate behavior, we condescend. Either way, we make sure we promote the incorrect actions.

Probably the greatest impact of the emotion of love is its ability to release an individual from the crippling and devastating emotion of fear. It is only when there is freedom from fear in a setting of joy and acceptance that a person is able to grow physically, mentally, and spiritually. This is well exemplified by the following words of the famous Indian poet Rabindranath Tagore: "Where the mind is without fear, the head is held high."

When an individual uses love as the basic emotion, no words are needed to convey it. The intent, actions, behavior, and attitude all reflect it. Say a child spills a glass of milk on some important papers. It is easy to get upset and use anger to guide our behavior and actions during that moment. But this only instills fear in the child, takes away a learning opportunity, and distances the child from the adult. On the other hand, when we have our actions guided by love, we want to use the event to teach the child to learn from mistakes and to find solutions. Anger promotes fear while love encourages understanding. Love actually serves as the most important motivational source toward progress, and yet it instills us with a sense of peace and well-being.

> *"In this life we cannot do great things. We can only do small things with great love."*
> ~Mother Teresa

Love is probably also the best reward that any child or adult can receive. When teenagers get the feeling of joy and acceptance from a family, they do not feel compelled to break norms to please their peers. A spouse will always be more agreeable when the undercurrent in an individual's tone is loving. A child is less likely to rebel or feel distressed if the adults in his or her life are understanding and loving. Dealings with colleagues or employees are unlikely to be difficult if we show acceptance and understanding toward them. In essence, all relationships of life are smooth, enduring, progressive, successful, and harmonious if the thread that weaves them is the fabric of love.

Studies on love and health have repeatedly shown that people who experience joy and acceptance are likely to have quicker recoveries, fewer complications, and lower mortality. Maybe there is some truth in the saying "Married men live longer...or at least it appears that way to them!"

Chapter 45

Bases of Harmony : Enjoyment & Appreciation

"The ideals that have lighted my way and time after time, have given me new courage to face life cheerfully have been Kindness, Beauty, and truth."

~Albert Einstein

Enjoyment or being engrossed in joy is a unique feeling of appreciation, happiness, and tranquility. It differs from pleasure, which is a sensation that pertains to a physical stimulus perceived and liked by an individual. We may feel pleasure when we see a movie on a big screen TV, but watching a funny movie, even if on a small screen, in the company of loved ones will be more enjoyable.

Moments of enjoyment are like beautiful designs chiseled into our hearts and souls that we can reflect upon and draw satisfaction from even later in life. These are not activities that need to be purchased by large sums of money; these are the small things in life that contribute to our sense of enjoyment; they are the music that an event plays on the strings of our soul. Walking by yourself in a beautiful, natural environment; playing with and listening to young, innocent children; and relaxing with your loved ones are simple examples of things that increase this incredible feeling in our lives. Try hugging a tree, lying on the grass, and gazing at the moon and stars. In fact, dependence on materialistic objects often takes over our senses so much that it tends to weigh down our feelings of freedom and enjoyment. As in the words of a famous British author,

"Every increased possession loads us with a new weariness."
~John Ruskin

When an individual learns how to enjoy, he learns to appreciate his living and nonliving surroundings. The next time you venture out for a walk, stop for a moment and look at a single flower. Note how each petal has been created to perfection, how pretty the color is, and how beautiful the supporting stem and leaves are. And then step back and look at the garden. Innumerable such floras smile back at you. The next time you interact with your children, note how wonderfully they have been created. Appreciate the brilliant questions they throw at you. Appreciate the fact that we are still alive on this beautiful earth, interacting with such wonderful people, surrounded by nature's immense beauty, and equipped with the wisdom to improve our and other people's lives.

That is the true magic of our lives—to appreciate and enjoy this world, each other, and the unseen power that guides us into balance. But the foremost emotion that should overwhelm us as we enjoy and appreciate is gratefulness. Just remember the times you wanted to go back and do more for someone who expressed gratitude to you for something you did. Nature is only going to bring you more as you appreciate and feel grateful for what you already have. It is pointless to be miserable about what you do not have if you cannot enjoy and appreciate what you do have to begin with. As the proverb goes, *"I cried because I had no shoes, till I met someone who had no feet."*

Chapter 46

The Strength of Soul— Sincerity & Service

When my ten-year-old daughter joined an after school program in which she provided care for small, needy children, I teased her about not spending enough time with her siblings. With complete sincerity she replied, "Mom, my brother and sister have everything: caring parents, all kinds of comforts, and much more. These poor children have hardly anything. It feels wonderful to be able to provide care, affection, food, and toys for these lonely kids." The sparkle in her eyes and the saintly expression on her face made me realize that this has to be a universal and ageless feeling. The feeling of serving with sincerity, asking for nothing in return, and drawing strength from the comfort of others is indeed a very satisfying experience.

Some people indulge in such activities for secondary gains: a way to be recognized, the goodwill associated with charity, etc. But true and sincere service is a reward in itself. Charity without the need to be recognized for it in the form of attending to another individual or living thing with only the other individual's needs in mind is the most supreme of all acts.

Mother Teresa, who served in the ruins of one of the neediest communities of Calcutta, was once asked how she felt about tending to the never-ending poverty. She promptly replied, "The spiritual poverty of the Western World is much greater than the physical poverty of our people". Her life truly exemplifies the uplifting, ecstatic feelings that this trait embodies. Her calling to serve the poor and needy came very early in her life, and in her words, she was given this calling "from the lord himself." Her life story serves as one of the most inspiring to me.

Only an individual who has tasted these enchanting, magical, majestic, and uplifting feelings is forever rich—rich with an inner strength, peace, harmony, bliss, and complete well-being.

Summary

If you lose your wealth, you have lost nothing,
If you lose your health, you have lost something,
But if you lose your character, you have lost everything.
~Woodrow Wilson

For most people struggling in this materialistic world, it is difficult to comprehend and accept this phenomenon. And yet this is the most important truth in our lives. A man who cannot be at peace within cannot find peace anywhere. And yet, the way we shape our health and character and bring ourselves into optimal physical, psychosocial, and spiritual health is in our hands. In the words of a famous German poet,

"The will of a man is his happiness."
~Johann Christopher Friedrich von Schiller

It is a paradox that we are fascinated by what constitutes the universe and yet do not care enough to know our neighbors and friends well! We expend an enormous amount of energy in exploring the world but do not have the time to gain knowledge about the details of our own bodies! We are curious about the discoveries that lie in the depths of the oceans and yet are ignorant of what is within us!

And as we explore our own depths, we are able to shape our own destinies. Destiny to me is the result of choices we make with the chances we are given. What has been provided in this book are the tools, techniques, ideas, and concepts that the author has gathered over nearly thirty years of learning in the medical profession and many more years in the experience of life. By simplifying these items for practical application, I have come up with nine essential steps for perfect health and complete well-being.[43]

- Believe that everything is there for a reason and live each day with a positive attitude.

- Keep the mind clear, allow only progressive thoughts, and promote useful habits.

- Live in the moment, be selective of your company, and find some time for yourself each day to enjoy a stress-free life.

- Eat a balanced diet with nourishing foods and plenty of fluids.

- Maintain a schedule for regular exercising.

- Ensure restful rest to rejuvenate daily.

- Feel peace by acknowledging the supreme power.

- Consciously evolve yourself to higher standards.

- Live in harmony by following the laws of nature.

In case doubt ever knocks on your door, remember the saying,

> *"Think you can, think you can't; either way you will be right!"*

---

[43]More information and updates are available on the website: URL- http://www.healthycenter.org

Part 2

Practicing the Nine Steps for Complete Health and Well-being

Preparing for the Practice

- *Arrange a check-up with your physician and undergo lab testing to rule out any kidney, heart, or endocrinal diseases that may prevent your ability to participate in fluid intake, exercises, or special diets.*

- *Follow each step until it has become a part of your daily life. This may take one day for someone, a week for another, and a month for yet another person.*

- *Remember: quick fixes only give short-term results. For lifetime health and well-being, one has to incorporate changes that will allow one to implement the right lifestyle.*

Step 1

Purify

The first step toward the achievement of health is to remove toxins from our systems. For the first week, simply concentrate on purifying the body through internal and external cleansing.

Internal Cleansing

- Ensure the intake of at least six to eight glasses of pure water by making a compulsory schedule. Start with one to two glasses of water every morning, take a glass or two of water before every meal, and be sure that the last thing you consume each day is a glass of water. Copy the chart on the next page and enter the times when water is consumed during the first week to establish the practice.

- Start minimizing any addictions that you may have developed by eliminating or decreasing the intake of the addictive substance.

External Cleansing

- Consciously begin washing or sanitizing hands before each meal and rinsing the mouth (if possible, even brushing the teeth) after each meal.

- Maintain a clean body and environment to enjoy a hygienic milieu.

Number of glasses of water	Mon	Tue	Wed	Thu	Fri	Sat	Sun
1							
2							
3							
4							
5							
6							
7							
8							

Step 2

Focus

The next step is to consciously live in the moment. Be fully aware of your surroundings, actions, and thoughts. Only when one is unconsciously thinking, do unnecessary thoughts start growing like weeds and taking over our happy and peaceful internal garden.

- Constantly strive to focus only on what is happening around you at any given time. The only real, truthful moment is this moment. The past does not exist anymore, and the future is pure anticipation. Life is now.

- At all times, try to remove any unnecessary subjective feelings that arise with a thought. These are often negative emotions that drain the strength of the mind, the soul, and eventually the body. Keep the mind and your environment free of clutter. Recognize and introduce positive influences in the form of happy and upbeat company, books, music, and TV shows.

- In order to avoid missing appointments, take time at the beginning and the end of the day to plan the day ahead. Keep an organizer handy that has a reminder alarm. A helpful organization chart to help you organize and plan for the week is given on the next page.

Time	Mon	Tue	Wed	Thu	Fri	Sat	Sun
7–8 a.m.							
8–9 a.m.							
9–10 a.m.							
10–11 a.m.							
11–12 p.m.							
12–1 p.m.							
1–2 p.m.							
2–3 p.m.							
3–4 p.m.							
4–5 p.m.							
5–6 p.m.							
6–7 p.m.							
7–8 p.m.							
8–9 p.m.							

Step 3

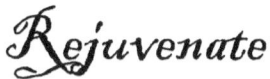

Rejuvenate

Just like our bodies need constant nourishment, our minds need to be rejuvenated and recharged on a regular basis. Donate fifteen to twenty minutes of your time each day to do this by meditation. This is the time during which you let all thoughts dissipate and you enter a peaceful state of pure bliss. (See section on Meditation-page 61).

This should ideally be done in the morning and evening, but whenever you have the time, sit in solitude in quiet surroundings and meditate, even if it is for just five minutes. Take a few deep and slow breaths and visualize energizing light filling your inner self and recharging you with peaceful and positive energy.

The following page pictorially depicts the states one might transcend to reach a rejuvenating mental and spiritual plateau.

Blissful State

⇑

Energizing Light

⇑

Thought-Free Mind

⇑

Subsiding Flow of Thoughts

⇑

Vibrating with Sound of "Aum"

⇑

Deep Breathing

⇑

Relaxed Body

Step 4

Nourish

Building and maintaining our bodies with the correct building blocks is clearly one of the most important steps toward healthy existence. Pay special attention to what and how you eat.

What You Eat

- Ensure the intake of at least two glasses of milk or an equivalent substitute, one of which should ideally be yogurt.
- Be generous in eating at least two servings each of thoroughly washed fresh vegetables and fruits.
- At least twice a day, eat a good protein source, such as eggs, legumes (including soy), fish, or lean meat.
- Eat cereal or bread made of whole grains instead of refined ingredients.
- Consume at least one serving of drink or food that is rich in antioxidants, such as tea, berries, pomegranates, or grapes.
- Eat a few nuts (almonds/walnuts) to provide omega fatty acids.
- Limit desserts to twice a week.
- Take supplements if needed (see page 119)
- Beware of and avoid toxins in the food or containers (see page 135)

How You Eat

- Find time to sit down and enjoy your food. Happy company helps!

- Chew the food well so that it is ground to a paste before you gulp it down.
- If possible, have designated times for meals and eat at regular intervals, ideally every four hours.

Breakfast	Glass of Milk/Yogurt
	Egg
	Whole-grain Bread/Cereal, such as Oatmeal
	Fruit
Lunch	Serving of Vegetables/Salad
	Lean Meat/Fish
Snack	Fruit and Nuts
	Antioxidant (berries/grapes/ pomegranate/tea)
	(My favorite: yogurt with berries/ raisins & walnuts)
Dinner	Serving of Vegetables
	Lentils/Soy
	Yogurt
	Whole-grain Bread/Tortilla

Healthy Eating

Step 5

Energize

Considering the innumerable positive effects that exercising has on health, keeping active should be absolutely essential for a healthy existence. It does not matter how much time one is able to put in; just starting the process is well worth the effort. Start with fifteen to twenty minutes a day for three days a week and gradually raise it to forty to sixty minutes a day for five to seven days a week.

Enhance Success

- Combine exercise with a fun activity, such as the company of a good friend, watching a comedy show, reading a humorous book, or walking in nature.
- Wear comfortable and appropriate shoes and workout clothing.
- Don't forget to breathe when exercising.
- Start slow and advance according to your level of tolerance.
- Drink adequate fluids.
- Try to incorporate the different types of exercise.

Types of Exercising

- Aerobic: At least thirty minutes three to five times a week.
- Stretching: At least twice a week
- Strengthening and Toning: At least twice a week

Aerobic

Walking

Jogging

Swimming

Tennis

Basketball

Stretching

Yoga

Pilates

Stretching exercises

Strengthening and Toning

Weight machines

Lifting weights

Yoga

Pilates

Step 6

Relax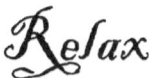

It is imperative that we find time daily to do things that give us joy and relaxation. These may be in the form of reading, watching TV, listening to music, meeting with friends, taking a warm shower, or getting a soothing oil massage. Additionally, setting up a routine that allows us to have restful sleep every night ensures recovery and vitality.

Stress-free Relaxation

- Play soothing music, CDs, or listen to comedic talk shows on the radio while driving.
- Invest in a treadmill and place it in front of TV and work out while watching a comedy show or movie.
- Find time for work-free interaction with happy friends.
- Plan a vacation to a fun place at least every six months.
- Indulge in body and face massage with aromatic oils once every month or every other month.

Ensuring Restful Sleep

- Keep a regular sleep time if possible.
- Ensure you have a comfortable mattress, pillow, and sheets on your bed.
- Minimize fluid intake for two hours and caffeine for six hours before bedtime.

- Keep your bedroom temperature comfortably cool and ensure the surroundings are noise free.
- Wash hands and feet and massage them with lavender/ sandalwood oil or lotion for a few minutes before sleep.
- Try milk and cereal or calcium and magnesium supplements if you have difficulty sleeping.

Relaxation
Music
Books
Comedy Shows/Movies
Happy Company
Massage

Sleep
Regularity
Physical Environment
Wind Down
Nutrition Before
Stress Free Mind

Step 7

Connect

Faith and hope are essential in life. Without them, there is bound to be undue distress and potential for depression. Connecting with the universal energies and powers to help put force in our own lives can only serve us well. By using the abundant proof of this energy around us, we can fortify our strength and belief.

Connect with Nature

- Once every day, take the time to looking at any natural, living thing, such as a tree, flower, or little animal, to realize how each organism has been created to perfection, provided for, and allowed to complete its life cycle with new, energized life by replacing other organisms that have completed their material existences.

- Enhance your knowledge of the universe to realize how the creation, sustenance, and recycling of the stars, planets, and life has been provided for to perfection by an unknown source of energy—the supreme power.

Connect with Spiritual Power

- Many spiritually advanced individuals, such as Mother Teresa, Mahatma Gandhi, and Martin Luther King Jr., have walked the face of earth. Their autobiographies serve as excellent sources of spiritual knowledge and enlightenment.

- Holy scriptures and religious texts can serve as additional support, but one should remember that all religions teach the same values and that interpreting them to enhance power, hatred, and violence is *not* spirituality, but the mere promotion of selfish, controlling ideas.

~

Supreme Power

Cosmos/Universe

Solar System

Earth

Living Beings

Humans

~

Step 8

Evolve

The history of the evolution of man is a testimony to the fact that progressive improvement in our development is capable of creating a masterpiece of pure potential and consciousness. It is only befitting to apply this to our own individual lives. Take a day or two to recognize the simple steps you can take toward each of the following steps of self evolution and attempt to incorporate them as daily habits.

Self Awareness

- Ask yourself "Who am I?" "What am I?" "What is my purpose on earth?" Investigate your true nature, character, and attributes. What are your worthy traits, and what needs to be changed?

Self Awakening

- Observe yourself as you conduct yourself alone and in the presence of other beings. What do you say and why? What do you do and why?

Self-Evolution

- With determination and effort, strive to raise your character and attributes to higher manifestations of spirit.

Evolve

⇑ <u>Effort</u>

Introduce Change

Awaken

⇑ <u>Observe</u>

Thought, Word, and Action

Aware

⇑ <u>Question</u>

Investigate Self

Self-Evolution

Step 9

Synchronize

The very purpose of life is to live in harmony with ourselves and our surroundings. Only by so doing can we enjoy complete peace, bliss, and a sense of achievement that is undeniably the most enriching experience possible. The wisdom given to us by observing the circle of life allows us to realize the virtues by which we can support and propagate the evolution of living entities. These virtues need to stay at the forefront of our conduct and may be summed up by the letters of the word *circles*, as given below:

C   Compassion- Treat others as you would like to be treated.

I   Intent and Action– Be Honest and hurt no one by monitoring your thoughts, words, and actions closely.

R   Respect- Treat yourself and others with dignity.

C   Creativity- Strive to bring into manifestation good images that linger in your imagination and let your talents unfold.

L   Love- Without judgment, unconditionally accept and rejoice with everyone, everything, and every situation.

E   Enjoyment and Appreciation- Take time to notice and express gratitude for all the wondrous creation around us.

S   Service and Sincerity- Spend some time serving without any selfish motives.

Ponder and strive to experience each of these states one day at a time.

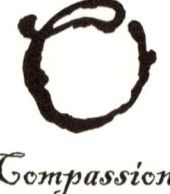

Compassion

Intent and Action

Respect

Creativity

Love

Enjoyment and Appreciation

Service and Sincerity

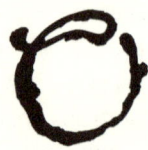

Synchronize with the
Circle of Life

Suggested Reading

Mind

As a Man Thinketh
By James Allen
Publisher: Grosset & Dunlap

The 7 Habits of Highly Effective People
By Stephen T. Covey
Publisher: Free Press

Don't Sweat the Small Stuff with Your Family
By Richard Carlson, PhD
Publisher: Hyperion

The Autobiography of Benjamin Franklin
By Benjamin Franklin
Publisher: Dover Publications

Best Organizing Tips
By Stephanie Winston
Publisher: Simon & Schuster

Love, Medicine and Miracles
By Bernie S. Siegel, MD
Publisher: HarperCollins

Psychology
By Charles G. Morris & Albert A. Maisto
Publisher: Prentice Hall

Practicing the Power of Now
By Eckhart Tolle
Publisher: New World Library

Ageless Body, Timeless Mind
By Deepak Chopra, MD
Publishers: Three Rivers Press

You Can Heal Your Life
By Louise L. Hay
Publisher: Full Circle

Don't Sweat the Small Stuff
By Richard Carlson, PhD
Publisher: Hyperion

Meditations for Women Who Do Too Much
By Anne Wilson Schaef
Publisher: Harper San Francisco

Body

Review of Medical Physiology
By William Ganong
Publisher: Appleton & Lange

Biochemical and Physiological Aspects of Human Nutrition
By Martha H. Stipaunak, PhD
Publisher: W.B. Saunders, Div. of Harcourt Brace and Company

Recommended Dietary Allowances
By National Research Council
Publisher: National Academy Press

Current Medical Diagnosis and Treatment 2005
By Editors Lawrence M. Tierney Jr.
Stephen J McPhee & Maxine A Papadakis
Publisher: Appleton & Lange

The Art of Yoga
By BKS Iyenger
Publisher: HarperCollins

The Encyclopedia of Healing Foods
By Michael Murray, N.D.
Publisher: Atria Books

Wheatgrass: Nature's Finest Medicine
By Steve Merowitz
Publisher: Sproutman Publications

Walking: The Ultimate Exercise for Optimum Health [Audiobook]
By Andrew Weil, M.D. and Mark Fenton
Publisher: Sounds True

Soul

Communion with God
By Neale Donald Walsch
Publisher: Berkley Books

Mother Teresa; Her Life, Her Work, Her Message
By Jose Luis Gonzale-Balado
Publisher: Liguori Publicatoions

Mahatma Gandhi; His life & Times
By Louis Fischer
Publisher: Bhavan Book University

Autobiography of a Yogi
By Paramahansa Yogananda
Publisher: Jaico Publishing House

The Holy Bible
Publisher: Good News Publishers

Peace in a Restless World
Chinmaya Publications

Meditations for Women Who Do Too Much
By Anne Wilson Schef
Publisher: Harper San Francisco

Bhagavad-Gita As It Is
By A.C. Bhaktivedanta Swami Prabhupada
Publisher: McPherson's Printing Group

Siddharta
By Hermann Hesse
Publisher: Bantam Books

Many Lives, Many Masters
By Brian L Weiss
Publisher: Simon & Schuster

Life of Pi
By Yann Martel
Publisher: Random House

The Gateway Experience (CD box set)
By Laurie Monroe
Publisher: Monroe Institute

Far Journeys
By Robert Monroe
Publisher: Bantam Doubleday Dell Publishing

The Five People You Meet in Heaven
By Mitch Albon
Publisher: Hyperion

Only Love is Real
By Brian L Weiss
Publisher: Simon & Schuster

Handbook for Mankind
By Buddhadasa Bhikkhu
Publisher: Thammasapa, Bangkok

www.ingramcontent.com/pod-product-compliance
Lightning Source LLC
Chambersburg PA
CBHW021547290526
45784CB00016B/79